KORE

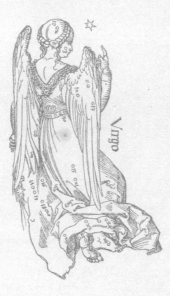

Andrzej Szczeklik

KORE

*On Sickness, the Sick, and the Search
for the Soul of Medicine*

Introduction by Adam Zagajewski
Afterword by John Martin
Translated by Antonia Lloyd-Jones

COUNTERPOINT
BERKELEY

Library of Congress Cataloging-in Publication is available.
ISBN 978-1-61902-019-1

Cover design by Nayon Cho for Quemadura
Interior design by Valerie Brewster after the original Polish edition

COUNTERPOINT
1919 Fifth Street
Berkeley, CA 94710

www.counterpointpress.com

Printed in the United States of America
Distributed by Publishers Group West

10 9 8 7 6 5 4 3 2 1

CONTENTS

Adam Zagajewski

INTRODUCTION

I first met Professor Andrzej Szczeklik in Paris in the 1990s when my principal personal identification document (as well as a Polish passport) was still a French *Carte de Résident*. This smiling, extremely sympathetic doctor made an excellent impression on me; we had only a short conversation, but at once I realized I was dealing with an unusual doctor and scholar, an experimental scientist and humanist all in one.

People who came from Krakow confirmed that I was not wrong; I heard about Szczeklik's famous clinic, where in the best possible conditions ordinary people were treated in addition to famous artists, including Czesław Miłosz. I understood that Andrzej Szczeklik is as much a good Samaritan as he is a brilliant academic. Soon after our return to Krakow, my wife and I were witnesses to an extremely amusing, cabaret-style launch for the Professor's book *Catharsis*. However, the book itself was serious; I was moved by its content, but also by the fact that the figure of the Author proved to be an extraordinary writer, combining sensitivity and humanist erudition with admirable expertise in the exact sciences (for, nowadays, medicine is this kind of science). I thought people like that had disappeared forever, and that we could only look back nostalgically into the past for universal authors who understand the life of the soul and the body.

I remembered that fifty years ago, in his famous lecture *The Two Cultures and the Scientific Revolution*, the British writer C.P. Snow fulminated on the fact that two spheres of learning (and education), the scientific and the humanist, had entirely parted company. He laid the blame at the door of the humanists (of course!).

I do not know who is to blame, or what the penalty should be, but the fact is, these two cultures have parted ways for good and all, and any author who tries to bridge this deep schism deserves attention and recognition. And if he does not try, we should be forgiving . . .

In past decades patients have often written about medicine; patients, or devotees of medicine such as the great Polish essayist Jerzy Stempowski, who was an amateur expert on pharmacology and medical procedures. In his beautifully written letters he occasionally imparted advice about health, or at least commented knowledgeably and sadly on the medical diagnoses given to his correspondents by professionals.

In some health care systems—in the United States, for example, where I have had occasion to seek a medical opinion—the doctor has changed into someone who appears before the patient for just a brief moment, like Zeus himself. The patient sits in a tiny little room with no windows, like a prison cell that has just been cleaned, and waits in solitude for quite a long time, until suddenly he hears a determined twist of the door handle, and there is God, in the person of a suntanned doctor, who asks two questions and then instantly vanishes. Before this revelation, and also after it, the patient is surrounded by an army of nurses—genial, jocular nymphs, but with no authority. Nowadays, the doctor's face is not so very different from a computer screen, or the cover of a journal such as *The Lancet* or *Nature*, or a checkbook . . .

So we are all the more interested in a writer who, like Andrzej Szczeklik, belongs to the ranks of the initiated, is a practitioner and theoretician, is familiar with human suffering, and knows all about the genome and other recent discoveries in the field of molecular biology. He is extremely well versed in the history of medicine, which includes not only the fates of geniuses and charlatans, and the clandestine theft of bodies needed by pathologists, but also the unusual observations that have led to breakthroughs in science. Nor does he ignore other, "soft" questions, doomed — just for now, or for all eternity? — to find no answer. Szczeklik writes with awareness of two kinds of problems: those that will one day be solved, and those that are sure to remain a mystery forever.

Humanists are often left helpless in the face of the big questions, but they could not manage without them. On the whole they regard representatives of the mathematical sciences with a touch of envy, knowing full well that in their own field there is not going to be any progress or sensational discovery for the world's press to write about. After all, the basis of the humanities (including poetry) is patient contemplation of the world and of art — a form of contemplation that does not involve any microscopes or X-rays, just the eye, the memory, and what Blaise Pascal called *l'esprit de finesse* (which is translated as "the intuitive mind").

What luck that we can still find an author who reads Dante, who understands — and shares — the disquiet of ancient and modern poets, who is so well read in the humanities, and who also helps us to comprehend the complexities of the most up-to-date medical theory. What a pleasure it is to read a book that succeeds in combining a competent discourse on modern biology with the intuition of an artist who knows that the physical health we need and desire so much, and that some of us so tragically lose, is not everything, because to be a human being means to ask questions about tomorrow, about the soul, about the meaning of life, and about infinity. In other words, to be a human being (even a healthy one, even a young one) is to be eternally dissatisfied, and to seek books that make a topic and a building material out of that dissatisfaction, thanks to which, paradoxically, they do something to assuage it. *Kore* is just this kind of book — it is Andrzej Szczeklik's very personal guide to medicine and the humanities, and also, to some extent, to his own recollections.

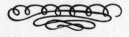

KORE

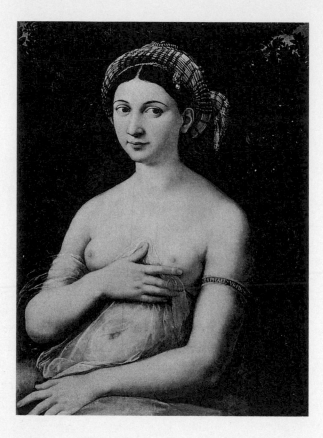

Raphael
La Fornarina, 1520
Galleria Nazionale d'Arte Antica, Rome

SYMPTOMS AND SHADOWS

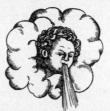

To tap and to listen, to look and to feel,
To make the eyes open and seek out the soul,
To hear out the breathing, to see fleeting clues,
To grasp just how simple the crux of it proves.

Coming home one evening, Raphael felt unwell and was seized by shivering and fever. Even though he had never known illness before, he sensed the approach of death. He received extreme unction and wrote his will, and a few days later he was no longer alive. He died on Good Friday, on his thirty-seventh birthday, at the height of his fame and universal adoration. Before dying, he said farewell to the woman he loved, entrusting her care to his faithful servant. He left us her portrait. Her name was Margherita, and she was known as La Fornarina, because she was the daughter of a baker (or *fornaio* in Italian).

From the picture a half-naked brunette looks out at us, her smooth raven-black hair wrapped in a turban. She has large black eyes and an inscrutable expression on her face. The light is falling from the right, and her gaze is most surely directed at the artist. There is a narrow gold and sapphire bracelet around her left arm with the name Raphael on it, "perhaps more than just the artist's signature." She has bared her breast and covered her belly in a veil, her hips in a pink skirt. Her pose is sensual and innocent all at once.

Behind her, against the black backdrop of the night, grows flourishing myrtle, the favorite plant of Aphrodite, goddess of love.

The woman's hand is resting on her naked left breast, with the fingers pointing towards the side of it and the armpit. If we follow this pointer, we might notice a slightly darker coloring at the edge of the breast, which is a very pale shade of blue. However, it is not a shadow, because the skin is drawn tight, bulging as if there is a lump, and so is the underarm area on the same side. If we take the analysis further by applying some special photographic techniques, it turns out that to render this bit of the portrait Raphael laid at least nine colors on top of each other, including some dark shades, while on the other side two colors were enough, pink and cream. A medical diagnosis was made for the first time in 2002, which declared that it was cancer of the left breast with probable metastasis to the axillary lymph nodes.

Was he the only one who knew? Or did she know too? Did they know what THIS meant? As the poet Czesław Miłosz says, THIS is like:

> *... the immobile face of someone who has just understood that he's been abandoned forever.*
>
> *Or the irrevocable verdict of the doctor.*
>
> *This. Which signifies knocking against a stone wall and knowing the wall will not yield to any imploration.*

Where do we get the bold idea of exposing the truth, casting THIS before the eyes of the world? It took the world four hundred and fifty years to notice and recognize Raphael's intention, though of course the accuracy of this medical diagnosis is debatable. It is not so much the actual diagnosis that comes into question as the fact that someone could go so far as to reveal sheer despair, so wholly and utterly—THIS.

The adored Raphael is buried in the Pantheon. His epitaph was composed by Cardinal Pietro Bembo, demonstrating the Renaissance style in all its splendor; in Thomas Hardy's version it reads: "Here's one in whom Nature feared—faint at such vying—/ Eclipse while he lived, and decease at his dying." These words echo with arguments that have been debated since Aristotle—whether art can only imitate nature, or whether, by creating it anew, it can master and perfect it. In Renaissance times and the centuries that followed, this argument about the boundaries of art also applied to the art of medicine.

What about La Fornarina, so greatly loved? The woman whose type of beauty appears in many of Raphael's works, in his most beautiful female figures? What was her fate? She was not allowed to take part in her lover's funeral because she was not joined to him by a church marriage. Only one bit of information has survived: an entry in the records of the convent of Sant' Apollonia in Rome dated 18 August 1520. On that day she crossed the threshold of the convent, and the gates closed behind her, never to reopen.

Historians of medicine tell us that, although women have suffered from breast cancer since ancient times, no description has been found that distinguishes it from other diseases of the mammary gland, neither in antiquity, nor for the next one-and-a-half millennia. Nor do we find it in Andreas Vesalius and Juan Valverde's wonderful Renaissance anatomical atlases, treasure-houses of medical symptoms. Only in the seventeenth century was a description of the clinical symptoms first published, enabling the differential diagnosis of breast cancer. And so Raphael noticed it one hundred years earlier, before the eyes of doctors had distinguished it from among a multitude of mammary gland conditions.

I have been looking at Raphael's work since birth. Above my parents' bed hung a medallion with a replica of his *Madonna*, and at the school I attended in Krakow, the Bartłomiej Nowodworski Lycée, which boasts an over four-hundred-year-old tradition of educating kings, poets and scholars, the ceiling in the vast entrance hall was covered in a fresco depicting *The School of Athens*. I do not think we ever had time to take a close look at it, neither in the mornings as we rushed to the start of classes at the last moment, nor in the breaks between lessons, as at the first sound of the bell we ran down the steps, through the theatrical hall and into the playground, where two games reigned supreme: soccer and *zośka* (also known as "footbag"). *Zośka* was played with a small, leaden metal ball, pierced in two places by a thin wire, with a woolen pom-pom attached to it to guarantee the airworthiness of this addictive toy as it was tossed by the foot. At the time we never gave any thought to *The School of Athens* or Raphael, or to the fact that in 1507 Pope Julius II invited him and some other renowned artists to renovate the Apostolic Palace. The visiting artists were sent to the Pope's private library, to a room known as the Stanza della Segnatura. After seeing only a few sketches by the twenty-four-year-old artist, the Pope was delighted, ordered the frescoes painted by the other artists to be "cast to the ground" and entrusted Raphael with the decoration of the entire apartment. Inside the *tondi* in the Stanza's vault we can see allegories of Theology, Philosophy, Justice and Poetry, linked to themes depicted on the walls. The fresco called *The School of Athens* corresponds to Philosophy. Inside a spacious, open building, crowned with mighty barrel vaults as a reference to

Donato Bramante's design for the new Saint Peter's Basilica, the philosophers are holding discussions in various groups. From the center of the picture two figures are walking towards us — Plato, with *Timaeus* in one hand and the other pointing to heaven, the transcendental seat of Being and the Idea; and beside him Aristotle, with his hand stretched ahead, between heaven and earth, to demonstrate that the Idea lies within the reality of the senses. A little lower, on one side of the steps, sits Pythagoras, surrounded by his pupils, presenting musical proportions, and on the other Euclid is leaning over a writing tablet with a compass in his hand, initiating some youths into the mysteries of geometry.

Only one man is dressed in contemporary clothing. We see him in the foreground, sitting on the steps, leaning his head on his hand; deep in thought, he is writing something in a notebook. This figure, identified with Heraclitus, is generally regarded as a portrait of Michelangelo in the years when the Sistine Chapel frescoes were being painted. He is wearing tall boots made of soft leather turned down below the knees. There are several lumps on his right knee. They look hard and compact, with no trace of redness or inflammation. To the doctor's eye they are a typical symptom of a distinctive disease. As we know that Michelangelo suffered from attacks of nephrolithiasis (kidney stones), we can accept with a high degree of probability that the lumpy growths on his knees are the hallmarks of podagra, in other words, gout. Lead could cause the disease to develop; it is said that while painting the Sistine Chapel he lived for weeks on end on bread and wine, which in those days was kept in lead vats.

And so illness showed its face to the eyes of a brilliant artist. More often, however, it stays hidden inside us, frightening us by remaining invisible. The doctor tries, briefly, to encourage it to reveal signs that he can use to build a diagnosis, define and name his adversary. The art of medicine depends *inter alia* on exposing the symptoms of disease. Just as a magician summons up spirits at a small, spinning table, so a doctor summons up the symptoms of an illness. But can we force an illness to drop its guard by tickling its foot? Yes, replied Joseph Babinski, and with this statement, based on his discovery of the so-called plantar reflex, he had a decisive influence on the development of neurology in the early twentieth century.

After making his discovery, Babinski presented the contemporary picture of neurology in a lecture addressed to the Royal Society in London. He began with a quotation from *Don Quixote*. One evening, after a long day of exhausting rambling, the knight errant stopped at the door of an inn. "Who's there?" shouted the publican, without turning the lock. In reply our hero presented his titles: "Duque de Béjar, Marques de Gibraleon, Conde de Bañalcazar y Bañares, Visconde de la Puebla de Alcocer, Señor de las Villas de Capilla, Curiel y Burguillos." The publican replied that to his regret he could not lodge so many people, and thereby deprived himself of a guest who might have procured him great profit.

The same sort of unfortunate episode, continued Babinski, awaits the student of medicine, as he tries to find room in his memory for the names of all the reflexes of the lower limbs. And here he reeled off about two dozen names that to spare the Reader we shall not mention. Admittedly, doctors had had a few hundred years to write down this long list of reflexes. They had begun to understand them thanks to Descartes, who was the first to comprehend what reflexes are—the automatic, stereotypical functions that do not involve "the intervention of our soul." And in a drawing showing a man retracting his foot from a blazing bonfire, he drew the path of a reflex: from the outer edge (the heel) to the central nervous system, and back to the muscle (the calf).

✦✦✦

Babinski owes his place in the history of medicine not so much to the fact that he brought order to a seemingly infinite number of limb reflexes, whose clinical value remained doubtful moreover, as to the discovery of the new symptom that bears his name. Retracting the leg in response to irritation of the sole of the foot had long since been familiar. Depending on the intensity of the stimulus, a dorsal bend of the foot was accompanied by a bend in the knee and the hip. No one paid any attention to the movements of the toes, nor were they ever mentioned in passing, until Babinski examined the response of the big toe to pricking or rubbing the sole, and noticed a difference between an upwards movement of the toe in disorders of the nervous system and a downwards movement among healthy people. He proved that this upwards movement, straightening the big toe, is an unusually sensitive indicator of disorders in the functions of the pyramidal system, along which all sorts of nerve routes run. He discovered what is in many people's view the most important of the symptoms that reveal disease of the central nervous system.

Joseph Babinski was born in Paris in 1857. His parents were Poles who had been forced to emigrate from Poland, and had met and married in France. His father, an engineer, even traveled to Peru for his work in order to secure a living for his young family. Not long after completing his studies, Babinski became first assistant to Jean Martin Charcot, who was at the height of his fame. Examining masses of disabled inmates at the Salpêtrière Hospital, including their brains and spinal cords whenever the chance arose, Charcot and his fellow workers identified many nervous diseases known to this day, such as multiple sclerosis. In 1890 Babinski left Salpêtrière to take the post of senior registrar in the neurology department at La Pitié Hospital, where he would continue to work until he retired thirty years later. Tall, statuesque and blue-eyed, "he had none of the typical Gallic *panache*." He would arrive at the hospital at nine-thirty by droshky, or in later years by car, with a taciturn chauffeur, change into a white tunic and proceed in silence to his consulting room, a converted four-bed hospital ward with chairs installed for his guests from France and abroad. He would sit with his back to the wall, within reach of a small table where his examination instruments lay: a neurologist's hammer, vibrating forks, a pincushion full of needles, test tubes containing hot and cold water and a stimulation apparatus using a constant or variable electrical current. Lined up in the corridor, the patients came in after entirely undressing behind a screen. Babinski would start by silently examining the patient, and then making some terse comments on his posture, gait and movements. After gathering a brief medical history, he would prompt a series of symptoms with the help of the hammer, needles or electrical stimulation, while an assistant noted down his laconic remarks. One day a dejected patient came to see him; once some galvanic electrodes had been applied to his temples he livened up, with his head bouncing now to one side, now the other, depending in which direction the current was flowing. Finally, Babinski completed the examination without saying a word. "Next!" he cried. But the amazed patient exchanged two words in a whisper with the nurse behind the screen and, just as he was, still naked, returned to Babinski's presence. Knowing that time is money, he asked one fundamental question. Pointing at the organ farthest from his head, located at the other end of his body, he asked: "Can't you find a way to liven that up a bit?"

Babinski deserves the credit not just for discovering the plantar reflex, but also for describing a whole gamut of symptoms that make up the whole of modern neurological semiology. His clinical demonstrations in the hospital amphitheater drew in crowds of people. Showered in the most prestigious international awards, he won fame in Europe and both Americas. "I am proud to have two motherlands," he said. "To one I owe my knowledge, and to the other the roots of my Polish soul." He asked to be buried in the Polish cemetery at Montmorency in the Paris suburbs. Towards the end of his life, he regarded his greatest achievement to have been paving the way for the first generation of French neurosurgeons. What he had succeeded in doing was to diagnose and precisely localize a tumor in the spinal cord, showing the neurosurgeon the exact spot where he should operate. He did this by pricking the back with his needles, finding sensation dysfunctions and observing the bending movements of the lower limbs. The master clinician had once again summoned up the spirit of the illness, diagnosed it and brought about a cure for the patient.

Before a doctor sets about the examination that we call objective — in other words, looking, feeling, tapping and listening — he talks to the patient, listens to his answers and gets to know the history of the illness. He helps the patient to "be free of forgetfulness." This is the root of the Greek word defining the truth, *aletheia*. Greek thought was permeated with the belief that the truth lives inside us. On the architrave of the temple at Delphi the ancients wrote: "Know Thyself," and like Plato they believed the truth is about remembering, or *anamnesis*. Meanwhile, to the truth itself they attributed a liberating force. In this sense the truth, as revealed by a patient telling a doctor his medical history, enables a diagnosis by being presented to the doctor. In almost half of all cases the diagnosis can be made from a skillfully gathered history of the illness. The rest is just its confirmation.

Sometimes it is hard for the patient to make himself heard. The doctor is in a hurry; he has his own worries, and simply isn't listening. Just like me, when at the age of seven my younger son Wojtek longed to have a tortoise. All his friends at school had either a cat or a dog, or at least a hamster, a guinea pig or a mouse. But he had no pets, and at home we refused to hear another word about that tortoise. Until finally ... When he was in second grade at elementary school he was given an assignment to write about: "The Animals at My Home." My son wrote a short piece, just one sentence: "At our house there are nothing but moths." That very day we bought him a tortoise. Only a week later, there were seven of them in the house. Dear Reader, in time of illness may you never have to resort to such extremes to have the doctor listen to you!

The situation can also be quite the opposite. Sometimes it is hard for the doctor to get through to the patient. Access is barred by lack of trust or a bad experience in the past. The patient remains closed within himself, behind a skin that you cannot force your way through — sometimes literally. I am doing my rounds. I approach a bed; the nurse draws back the quilt and shows me a powerfully built man. His entire body is covered in tattoos, from his neck to his toenails. There are naked figures of women festooned in adages and elaborately swirling lines of poetry — all in Latin, throbbing with meter. I lean closer and find Ovid's *Ars amandi* and *Metamorphoses*, and then Horace's *Odes*. I am reading my school lessons from decades ago on this man's skin.

Our patient has recently come out of jail, where he spent two years in a cell with a doctor of classical philology who worked on his body. I put my stethoscope to his heart, and there I find Horace: *Mutato nomine de te fabula narratur* ("Change the name and the story is about you"). *Nomen, nominis*, I am thinking — which declension is that? Third or fourth? I am not sure, and I cannot concentrate. The rhythm of the hexameter starts to obscure the rhythm of the heart. "I'll come and see you later," I tell the patient. He shows no surprise. Naturally, I want more time to admire his tattoos.

There are also some illnesses that play the diagnosis to the doctor themselves, like the Aeolian harp. Here comes a digression:
the harp, as we all know, is one of the oldest instruments. It was
played in Assyria and Babylonia, and in Greece and Rome too, of
course. However, nowhere has it ever been as exalted as it is in Ireland, where it was made the state emblem. You would have to love
poetry and music to ignore the lion or any other predator and make
a choice like this one instead. Ireland has given the world some
great poets. One of them, Seamus Heaney, noticed the similarities
between Poland and Ireland and said that in a way both countries
are the invention of poets and romantic musicians! Developing this
blatantly paradoxical idea, he added: "In both countries, the preservation of cultural memory and the ideal of national independence
were mutually fortifying projects."

The Aeolian harp first appeared at the end of the seventeenth
century and gained popularity in the Romantic era, because it was
especially dear to the Romantics — they felt a spiritual kinship with
it. Set up in gardens and parks, in courtyards and on palace roofs,
it awaited its musician. However, it wasn't played by a person,
but by gales and storms, winds and hurricanes. Thus it was heard
whenever the elements were aroused, "when the spirit appearing in
nature or present within it felt the desire to speak aloud." The Polish poet, Juliusz Słowacki, especially in his epic poem *Beniowski*,
made it an element of many similes, equating his entire "native
country" with it:

> ... *and further Podolia*
> *Houses and copses, the beehives, the song thrush*
> *Playing like harp strings, just made for this purpose*
> *By aged Aeolus.*

In yet another canto the statue of a poet "made out of sylla-bles"—his entire poetic work—is compared to the Aeolian harp:

Round him a forest of cypress and larches,
He will groan forth, like the harp of Aeolus.

Our vocal cords are no match for the number of strings on an Aeolian harp. We only have two of them inside us to pro-duce sound. But in illness they start to vibrate, plucked by a vio-lent movement of air as our lungs start to feel a lack of it. This is the music of breathlessness. Whenever a patient who is having an asthma attack comes into the consulting room, the wheezing so typical of this illness can be heard with the ear alone, heralding its onset. It is soon joined by whistling, and the stethoscope reveals continuous sounds, called rhonchi, above both lung fields. Wheez-ing and whistling are technical terms that a medical student comes across in his first years of study. After all, the wind makes a chim-ney whistle, and air makes an accordion wheeze. Air from the lungs is sent into a turbulent spin that is alien to it, jostles the contracted walls of the bronchi, making them shudder, and tugs at the vocal cords—like the strings of an Aeolian harp. In another disease, pul-monary edema, the air has to force its way through fluid that sud-denly starts to fill the tiny alveoli; above the rib cage characteristic crackles, called rales, can be heard, which tell us about an extreme danger whose critical moment will occur in less than twenty min-utes. Is it any surprise that the ancient Greeks were afraid of the winds too, especially the ones that raged across the world under the command of Boreas, enveloped in a storm cloud? They mud-dled people's minds, swept them away and assaulted women. Until finally Zeus and Poseidon carved out a labyrinth of caves and tun-nels on a desert island and imprisoned all the winds in them. And only in time of need did Aeolus, son of Poseidon, smash the surface of the rocks with his trident to set one of the prisoners free, and then stop up the opening. He even gave the winds to Odysseus for his journey in a sealed sack, but Odysseus's companions did not make good use of them.

Poland has a mountain wind called the *halny*, which is one of the kind that "carries in it the seeds of madness." A day or two earlier a silence sets in, the air stands still, and an overpowering heat beats down from a clear blue sky, with just a flat bank of clouds settling above the peaks of the Tatras. Then the *halny* strikes. The wooden highland houses creak and sway ominously, and spruces on the slopes snap like matchsticks, hillside after hillside. People are overcome with fatigue and depression, and black thoughts come to mind. Not everyone can withstand it. After two days we sometimes hear that someone or another—strangely, it is usually a local person—has hung himself. Just as in faraway Catalonia, where the *tramontana* strikes. The *halny* is from a family of warm, southern mountain winds, and in the Alps it is called the *föhn*. It is a wind of equally fatal consequences as the ones that strike the western islands on the Irish coast and "drive the sunniest natures into depression and bring with them an avalanche of acts of violence and suicides." Right up until the 1820s, when the *föhn* was blowing in central Switzerland it was unlawful for tribunals to assemble.

It would be futile to expect medicine to explain the strange effect of these winds on the human organism. It can cope much better with the "pulmonary winds" that are born inside us.

Modern technology has produced some formerly unknown opportunities to listen to them, and even to cure them from a distance. One of my patients, who is very well attuned to herself, was on a trip abroad when she started having coughing fits and breathlessness. She read everything she could find about paroxysmal coughing on the Internet and, by pressing a computer key, listened to a huge range of different coughs recorded in an electronic encyclopedia, and then made her own diagnosis. Then she recorded her coughing on a CD, sent it to me by courier and asked for my diagnosis. What could I do? I confirmed her self-diagnosis and prescribed some safe drugs over the phone. It worked! Although, as sometimes happens in medicine, there remained a doubt whether the cough that had been examined in such a modern way had not simply cleared up on its own!

But not everything runs like clockwork in medicine. There are some illnesses that play games with the doctor, teasing him maliciously and having fun leading him up the garden path. The rare illness of which I am now thinking, pheochromocytoma, is known as the great imitator. It takes a variety of symptoms from other conditions and displays them in its own sweet way, as if to play tricks on the doctor, his skill and his knowledge, to thumb its nose at him. It sows confusion in the minds of doctors, which soon changes into doubt. But as a young doctor at the start of my career at a hospital in Wrocław, I became convinced that this was exactly what I was dealing with in one of my patients. I was ready to nail it, to pin it down. I elaborated an entire argument, churned out the evidence in writing and discussed it with our radiologist. To catch and expose the illness, his help was essential. In the days when I began my clinical practice, ultrasounds were unheard of, as were computed tomography and magnetic resonance imaging — but by using a strange technique, introducing liters of air under the lower back behind the peritoneal cavity, the radiologist could try to reveal a small suprarenal tumor, which in my view was the perpetrator of the illness. Doctor Stanisław K., an experienced radiologist, a tall, thin, taciturn man with a kind heart, created the artificial pneumo-peritoneum and took some pictures. He stared and stared at the plates, until finally he pointed a finger and said: "Do you see? Just here. I think you're right." That meant it was necessary to operate.

On the morning of the operation I was at the radiologist's office early. I was quivering with anxiety. Was it absolutely for certain? Could we be wrong? I was still waiting for one more confirmation from the lips of my senior colleague, a renowned specialist. But Stanisław K. was silent for a long time, until finally he said: "Doctor Szczeklik, don't look to me for certainty. Radiology is the science of shadows." So were we like Plato's prisoners, shackled at the bottom of a deep cave, where they can only see shadows flickering on the walls? Were we mistaking those shadows for reality? And was that all we could see, those of us who were not free of "the fetters of the world of appearances"? There was a buzzing noise in my head, and the whole world was going dark. Put off my stride, feeling very anxious and unconfident, I headed for the operating theater, dragging my feet like a prisoner in chains, with the long thin shadow of my radiologist cast ahead of me as we went to face Professor Wiktor Bross.

This illustrious surgeon was a hotspur, famous for his sudden bursts of anger. That day there were flashes of lightning blazing from his diminutive figure. We were all afraid of him. But he seemed to fear nothing and no one. Without turning a hair, he would tackle operations that were bristling with dangers, confirming his place as Number One in the virgin territories of surgery. He had no doubt about it. He was only occasionally rattled when the outstanding Łódź heart surgeon, Professor Jan Moll, was mentioned in his presence. But it was always a passing cloud, just a small one that instantly dispersed, and with it the temporary anxiety over who was the front-runner, who was in the lead, who really was the best.

The first time I ever saw him was during summer student practice, making his rounds of the patients. His progress through the large neo-Gothic hospital ward was like a storm, with the professor leading the way, followed half a pace behind by the matron, and then the associate professors, junior professors, assistants, volunteers and students. As the long snake of figures in white was winding its way between the beds, the students at its tail were still stuck in the corridor. There was no time for a patient to get undressed once the professor was standing over her — that would have caused a burst of anger, which was why a ward sister ran ahead before the round as a vanguard, rushing from room to room and calling out to the patients: "Panties off! The professor is coming!" It was to face this person — fearless but terrifying in his anger — that we were now going.

The professor received us with refined politeness, and invited us to scrub up together. As the operation went ahead, I admired his virtuosity, steady-handedness and speed. However, time began to move very slowly for me when the professor started searching for the tumor in the open belly. "I can't feel anything here," he said loudly. "And why can't I feel anything? Why can't I find anything? Because there's nothing here!" he answered himself with rising satisfaction, getting into an effervescent mood. He went on making fun of us, quite mercilessly, and I felt as if time had come to a complete standstill. Until finally . . . "A chance discovery," he said, digging out the suprarenal tumor we had been looking for, which was the size of a pea. "I doubt very much if this has anything to do with the illness," he added. But we — and by now there was nothing but shadows left of us — sighed with genuine relief.

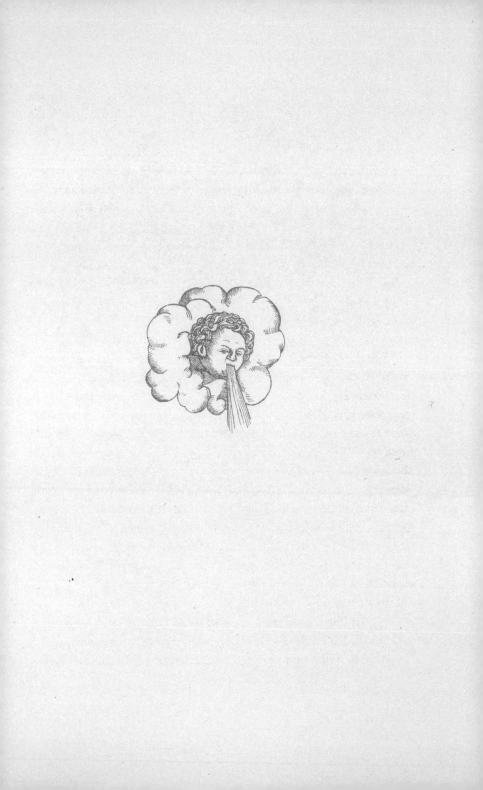

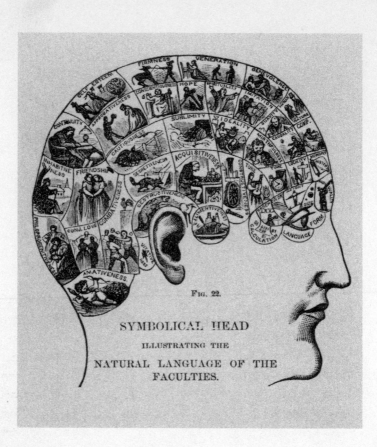

An Illustration from *How to Read Character. A New Illustrated Hand-Book of Phrenology and Physiognomy, for Students and Examiners; with a Descriptive Chart*, New York 1891

ABOUT THE BRAIN

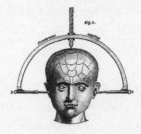

It was like the huge ball of cassata ice cream my mother had brought into the kitchen years ago and put in a deep plate, where it sat waiting to be served at table that evening. Now, in the same kitchen, in an identical soup plate, lying before me — smooth, shiny and egg-shaped, in a fine mist of formalin vapors — was a human brain. I had smuggled it out of the mortuary after our practical anatomy class. On the way home it had quivered in a plastic bag like a live fish bought for the traditional Polish Christmas dinner and, being equally slippery, it had very nearly slithered from my hands as I transferred it to the plate. Although I had followed, as it were (though quite unconsciously), in the footsteps of the great doctors and painters who had even managed to steal bodily remains from graveyards in order to study them carefully at home, I was not in fact driven by their unquenchable curiosity, but rather by fear of an approaching test on the anatomy of the brain. Shrouded in a menacing aura, this test was supposed to be the hardest obstacle to surmount in the first year of medical studies. "With your brains you'll never get through the brain test!" our junior lecturer had scornfully declared, rubbing his hands together. As I stared at the smooth surface of the large hemispheres, covered in grooves and furrows, at the folds of flattened, twisted coils, and imagined everything that lay hidden beneath them, I thought with rising terror that maybe the junior lecturer was right.

Fortunately, centuries before me, others had not given in to their horror at the sight of the brain, but had tried to understand it, ascribing definite functions to its mysterious though clearly separate areas. And so Franz Joseph Gall retained the childhood impression that people with goggle eyes typically have an excellent memory. Years later, as a young Viennese doctor, he thought that perhaps other features of the mind could have their seat in the brain and could shape its surface as they underwent either hypertrophy or atrophy. So as "the skull fits the brain like a glove," all these bulges or depressions in the brain should find their reflection in it. And he claimed that by feeling the skull bones you could discover a person's intellectual and moral characteristics. He provisionally defined twenty-seven bumps on the skull that were supposed to correspond to features such as courage, sociability, cantankerousness, pride, arrogance, parental feelings, artistic abilities, criminal or abstract tendencies and others. As you leaf through the catalog of these features, which grow in number with the course of time, the entry "love" never appears among them. It is not born in the brain, but rules over it.

Gall's theory, known as phrenology, had incredible success. It was already gaining renown in 1807 when the Austrian emperor banned its practice as at variance with the Catholic religion, because it promoted the belief that spiritual life had been proved to have a material nature. At this point Gall moved to Paris, from where his circle of adherents quickly spread about Europe. In Great Britain in 1832 there were already twenty-nine active phrenology societies regularly publishing at least a dozen periodicals. However, phrenology flourished first and foremost on social ground, because detecting the bumps on each other's skulls provided favorable conditions for flirtation. However, that does not mean it dropped its scientific packaging. In a print dated 1907 we see a young woman being examined by an electric phrenometer. She is standing on a high pedestal with her head in a glass dome, as if she were at the hairdresser's. A network of wires links the dome to a measuring machine the size of a person, with a glazed interior full of levers, gears, shafts and cogs. All this impressively complicated clockwork machinery is revealing and registering the intellectual features reflected in her skull. The woman is aware how serious the situation is; her focused expression shows a mixture of fear and anticipation at the revelation of the truth.

Francis Crick, the joint discoverer of DNA, remembered his mother taking him as a child to see a phrenologist. In Great Britain the last phrenology societies ceased to operate in 1967, and to this day in London antique stores you can find small porcelain heads with character traits and dispositions marked on them. For all his charlatanry, Franz Gall was a superb anatomist. He explained and described the routes of the major nerves from the cortex to the spinal cord. Malicious tongues say that today we are once again letting ourselves get carried away on a wave of neophrenology. Using a positron spectrometer, it beguiles us with images of the thinking brain—in false colors—prompting the belief that we are able to understand the computational techniques used to create such images.

Gall's concept that certain areas of the brain hemispheres correspond to defined functions proved in essence to be true. Let us imagine we are faced with a patient who has suddenly lost his power of speech. He is conscious, he can move about freely, and he can understand what we are saying to him, but he cannot say anything, and he replies to every question with two meaningless syllables, "bla-pa." We diagnose motor aphasia. In the mid-nineteenth century some Parisian doctors first drew attention to this unusual form of illness, and in the case of several affected patients they then described degenerative changes in the brain discovered at the autopsy. They were usually shaped like a small bladder the size of a quail's egg and were full of fluid. They always occupied one and the same place in the frontal lobes, to be more precise, in the *gyrus frontalis inferior*. They were also always found in the left hemisphere. This was reckoned to be an accidental coincidence. Finally, the observations covered at least a dozen patients. The idea that the center of speech, as it began to be called, could be located in only one hemisphere sounded sacrilegious, because it broke the taboo about the symmetry of the brain hemispheres. And at the time doctors already had a reverential approach to manifestations of symmetry, running ahead of contemporary physicists in this regard by more than a century. Meanwhile, the number of observed cases was rising; the changes were invariably on the left side. And finally during an autopsy an identical "bladder" was noticed, situated in exactly the same place as had always been described before, but in the right hemisphere. However, the patient whose brain showed this aberration had never suffered from aphasia. At this point Paul Broca, whose name was later to christen the center of speech, said: *Nous parlons avec l'hémisphère gauche* ("We speak with the left hemisphere").

Broca, a Parisian doctor, kept the brains of his first patients for posterity. After preserving them in formalin, he donated them to a museum in Paris. In 2007 some American neurologists took them out of the museum and examined them using magnetic resonance imaging. They confirmed the accuracy of Broca's observations. The center of speech occupied the area he had defined, slightly bigger than in the simplified version passed on by his successors.

Despite outward appearances, like all other vertebrates, we are built asymmetrically. We have our heart on the left side and our liver on the right. The embryo that results from the union of a sperm and an egg cell still has some features of symmetry. But it soon gives way, in the first stages of embryonic development. In the human embryo, consisting of a few dozen cells, the gene that corrugates its uniform surface (known as the "notch gene") becomes active, giving it a hallmark, a single, isolated feature, located on the left side of the embryo. Thus asymmetry is born long before a human being is born. After only a few days, the right side of an embryo is already distinct from the left. And so we could say that in the mother's womb we find a reflection of the breakdown of symmetry that occurs when a universe comes into being. Indeed, it breaks down in a similar way in a fraction of the first second of the Big Bang, bringing spherical symmetry down to "an orbital state," a point concentrating all matter. The fate of the universe is determined in that break.

The asymmetry of the cerebral hemispheres is revealed when we cut the big bond (the corpus callosum) that unites them. This bridge, made up of over two million nerve fibers, joins the hemispheres together and synchronizes their work. In the 1960s it was quite often destroyed entirely, surgically bisected in patients suffering from the most severe forms of epilepsy to prevent the transfer of discharges from one hemisphere to the other. In the early stages of reconvalescence the symptoms of splitting the brain were striking. The right hand reacted differently from the left to questions about numbers. Clinical anecdotes feature patients who buttoned up their pajama tops with one hand, but unbuttoned them with the other. After this temporary phase the symptoms passed off, and the patients talked, behaved and felt the same as before the operation. And yet closer examination revealed a profound split-brain syndrome. One hemisphere, on receiving information, was found not to share it with the other. And so it was recognized that patients with a split brain have "two conscious minds."

Diagnostic imaging conducted on healthy people supported these clinical observations, indicating that in most of us the left hemisphere specializes in speech, writing and reading, while the right one is dumb. As a result, the right hemisphere sometimes came to be called the lesser, redundant one. Yet in fact it contains some specialized centers of perception that are absent on the other side, such as the ability to recognize faces.

The selectivity of brain injuries is astounding. For example, carbon monoxide poisoning can cause cognitive malfunctions. They manifest themselves as an inability to distinguish colors (achromatopsia), a loss of perception of motion (akinotopsia) and an incapacity to recognize faces (prosopagnosia), among others. For almost a hundred years they were defined as "soul blindness" (*Seelenblindheit*). This term seems to have its origin in Plato, because the founder of the Academy ascribed a cognitive function to the soul — either directly or with the help of the senses. His view came down through the centuries and finally settled in medicine, until Sigmund Freud rechristened the poetic term with the more concise and scientific word "agnosia." And the soul vanished from symptomatology.

One time a middle-aged man was brought to our intensive care unit who had suddenly had a brain hemorrhage. He was in a deep coma, and for three weeks a respirator breathed for him. Then his own breathing returned, he began to react to pain and voices, gradually he started to perform the simplest functions and finally he could carry out simple instructions. One morning on my rounds I rather automatically asked him: "Good morning, Jacek, how was your night?" and he fluently replied: "Good morning, Jacek, how was your night?" and then repeated it twice more in one go. So he answered like a parrot, which doctors tactfully call "echolalia." It was like that for several days, until the echolalia passed and the first independent words started to emerge from him. He spoke in telegraphic style, in the simplest phrases. But now we could communicate. We asked him to write down a few words. He held the pencil over the paper for a long time, and then gave it back in a flustered state. Nor could he read the newspapers, not even the headlines. We diagnosed alexia and agraphia (loss of the ability to read and write). The next day, an excited nurse called me over to him. He was lying there reading a book! In Latin! It was a textbook for learning Latin that a medical student had left by his bed. Our patient, a professor of classical philology and a great expert on Ovid, had instantly got down to reading it. And then he wrote us several quite long sentences in Latin. Wanting to answer him, we summoned the help of the chaplain. Two months later the patient left the hospital unaided. He could talk, falteringly, with pauses, though understandably, but he was only just learning to read and write in Polish again. He could read and write fluently in Latin!

Similar language confusions, though extremely rare, have been described in Japan, where two kinds of symbol are used in writing. *Kanji*, the ideograms adopted from Chinese, represent whole words. Much later on *kana* were introduced, phonograms that reflect the sounds of vowels or consonants. The educated Japanese knows thousands of *kanji* by heart, though there are only seventy-one *kana* signs; modern writing is a mixture of *kanji* and *kana*. The patients were described as having aphasia of Broca's speech center (such as characterized our patient too), and had lost the ability to read and write in *kana*, though they could manage superbly in *kanji*. Reverse cases were also recorded, where the patient could read and write fluently in *kana*, but had total agraphia and alexia in *kanji*.

Alongside Broca's area, other centers gradually began to emerge. They were discovered during neurosurgical operations, when the surgeon, wanting to be sure about the vitality of the tissue surrounding the tumor he was removing, would gently stimulate it with an electric current, and the patient would respond with a movement of the body. The sensory zones also proved accessible in cases in which patients undergoing an operation had come out of the initial anesthetic applied while exposing the cortex, and could not then feel any pain while the brain was being stimulated, but, fully conscious, could describe their sensations. And so, on the basis of the body's responses, gradually a map of the brain was drawn. The first continent was located around the fissure of Rolando, the furrowed cleft running centrally from the top and dividing the cortex into two areas. In front, in the twists directly adjoining it, lie the motor zones, while at the back are the sensory zones. The former set individual parts of the body in motion, while the latter receive sensory impressions from them. They are symmetrical in relation to each other, though the proportions of the body to which they correspond have been shaken up, becoming almost grotesque. They reflect the sensitivity and discriminatory abilities of the individual parts rather than their size. In anatomical atlases they are often represented as two little people lying on the brain on either side of the fissure of Rolando. The surfaces occupied by their torsos and legs are relatively small, while the areas corresponding to the tongue, lips and fingers are huge. Moreover, the bodies of these homunculi look as if they are badly put together; for example, the face is not joined to the head and neck, but appears just under the palms of the hands. In animals the layout is similar, though the proportions are different: in the rat a huge area is occupied by the cortex that controls the whiskers, and in pigs the snout. We receive sensation in this area of the brain as a touch, a tingling or pinching feeling and thus as elementary, surface impressions. The seats of the refined, higher feelings should be sought elsewhere, beyond the twists surrounding the fissure of Rolando.

Before we come to them, let us mention one more famous brain operation that is usually associated with the beginning of modern research on memory. In 1957 an operation was performed on a twenty-seven-year-old man, H.M., to remove large pieces of the temporal lobes on both sides and adjoining fragments of the hippocampus, as a last resort against incurable epilepsy. The illness did indeed subside, but it took the patient's memory with it. He did not know what had happened several years before the operation, and quickly forgot current events. If someone left the room and came back a few minutes later, he could not remember ever having seen that person before. An hour after a meal he was unable to say what he had eaten, or whether he had eaten anything at all. Yet he was conscious, still had his short-term memory of events up to a few minutes ago and could fluently answer questions about current circumstances. What he had irreversibly lost was his "long-term, declarative memory."

Shortly afterwards, some even more acute memory dysfunctions were described in the case of a brilliant musician. He survived a viral infection of the brain that almost killed him, leaving both temporal lobes permanently injured. He still had a foggy idea of who he was, but he could no longer learn anything. Only his superior musical abilities remained unaffected. He lived the rest of his life in the present time; he had no childhood or past. "Like an actor in a Greek tragedy, he moves through life, unaffected by events around him, impervious to the passage of time."

How (if at all) does a person's psyche change after a cerebral stroke? When he regains consciousness weeks later, and then months or years later the power of speech, is he still himself? And if he isn't, who is he? What a test for our "self," which we intuitively accept as something unchanging, as the core that determines who we are! But is that right? And especially after such a serious illness, do we not become someone else, just in the old packaging? The great author and playwright Sławomir Mrożek asks about this in his recent book. He suffered a severe cerebral stroke with aphasia, and lost the ability to use the Polish language in speech or writing. He did not know how to count or converse in any language. In addition, the aphasia limited his ability to distinguish opposing concepts such as left and right and his capacity to determine distance and time. After almost three years of working with a speech therapist he could talk and write, and had regained his lost abilities. The final result of the therapy was *Baltazar*, his autobiography, in which his perfect memory of the details is striking, and so is the clarity of past events.

Baltazar was the writer's new name; apparently he learned this in a dream. It reminds us of the last ruler of Babylonia, whose end was predicted by a mysterious inscription that appeared on the wall during a feast: *Mene, mene, tekel, upharsin*, that is: "counted, weighed, divided." In dreams the veil obscuring a deeper reality is lifted and a person comes into contact with some mysterious forces. It is amid his dreams, in the "epic poem of the night" — *Forefathers' Eve* by Adam Mickiewicz — that Gustavus changes from a lover overcome by longing for personal happiness into Konrad, the man for whom the national cause is his life's focus. *Gustavus obiit — hic natus est Conradus.* We express our identity with a first name and a surname. Sławomir Mrożek writes that ever since he changed his name and has signed himself "Baltazar," "no one can either praise or criticize me any more for anything I wrote before the aphasia, because that person no longer exists." In my opinion his autobiographical book belies that statement, because "what makes us whole is memory and speech."

The question of identity is starting to crop up unexpectedly in transplantology. It certainly was not anticipated in 1952, when the first kidney was transplanted, or in 1967 after the first heart transplant. Until recently, almost all transplants involved internal organs, hidden inside the recipient's body. It was only visible transplants — of the hand or face, for example — that brought up questions of identity.

In 2005 French surgeons transplanted a large part of the face of a young woman — skin, subcutaneous tissue, muscles and even bits of bone. The operation was successful, the patient regained the ability to swallow and her speech improved, though her facial expression remained extremely handicapped. The novelty of this procedure, apart from the extent of the actual operation, was the fact that for the first time ever virtually a whole face was taken from the corpse of another woman. And so there was no previous transplant to compare with this one, because the face is the mirror of our identity and personality. How does a person feel when she is *wearing* someone else's face instead of her own? Who does she see in the mirror? How does the donor's family feel as they look at the face of their beloved relative "transplanted" onto a stranger? In such cases medicine is starting to talk of an "identity split." It does not have to be the face; a hand is enough. A New Zealander who had a hand transplant with very good results soon began to regard it as something alien; he could not bear the sight of it, stopped taking his immune-suppressant drugs and finally insisted on an amputation. He preferred to live without a hand than with a split identity.

It must be the memory that determines identity. For the Greeks, memory was also the mother of all the Muses: *Mnemosyne mater Musarum*. And if "distance is the essence of beauty," because only distance purifies the reality of what Schopenhauer called the "will-to-life," which is the source of suffering, of all our overwhelming possessive desires, then distance is achieved when the world appears in our memories. This "bountiful memory, one twinned with Imagination," sets before our eyes vivid images, rich in details, not pale, languid shadows. However, it does not come running to report at our command. To recover time gone by, to summon up the past with an effort of will is sometimes a futile exercise, because the past can be hidden beyond the reach of the intelligence "in some material object, which we do not suspect." And only chance decrees whether or not we shall encounter it. For Marcel Proust, the small sponge cakes called madeleines were just such a material object. Dipped in tea or a lime flower tisane, they evoked memories of childhood and brought happiness. They caused a revelation, an epiphany. In this simultaneous experience of the present and the past, Proust began "to see clearly in a state of rapture."

There can also be pain and suffering lying in wait for us in our memories. For fear of reviving them, we prefer to "turn years, whole periods into a void, a vacancy." For hell, in Czesław Miłosz's view, "is big screens showing films from our memory" — just as in Stanisław Lem's novel *Solaris*, where the mysterious, omnipotent Ocean surrounding the space station invades the minds of its inhabitants to find whatever is buried deepest in their memories. It creates an incarnation of figures from the past, each of whom is a source of terrible remorse, causing despair, shame and madness.

There is no way to rid yourself of these spectral emanations, these phantoms — you cannot even catapult them into outer space. And "One need not be a chamber to be haunted, / One need not be a house; / The brain has corridors surpassing / Material place." Sometimes a shocking memory, outwardly stripped of all connotations, is prompted by a trivial occurrence. One afternoon we were sitting having tea with a few guests, when the cat came into the living room. The woman sitting next to me went cold and pale, and from her lips that had suddenly gone blue there came a desperate cry: "Take away that monster this instant!" A similar case of sudden, panic-stricken fear at the sight of a cat was described in his journeys by the amazed Herodotus. In what depths of the brain is this painful memory preserved? How has it survived through generations, to utter the same cry thousands of years on?

I was once asked to examine an eminent professor of the history of literature, whose behavior had started to concern his relatives. We began our conversation. He spoke interestingly, brilliantly, just as I had imagined him years ago when as a student I had read his essays on Marcel Proust, among other writers, with excitement and admiration. It was not hard to steer the conversation onto that subject, onto the passage of time, and time lost. And once we were immersed in the topic of time, I asked: "Professor, could you draw a picture to say what time it is?" He showed no surprise, took a piece of paper and a pencil, but soon after when he handed them back to me, I saw an empty clock face, with the hands of the clock next to it. The page he had handed me gave me the diagnosis — Alzheimer's disease. His memory was disintegrating, and with it the entire world was collapsing into disconnected parts.

How could I fail to mention Ronald Reagan at this point? And the memorable words with which, about fifteen years after the end of his second term, the former president — conscious of his progressive, unstoppable Alzheimer's disease — addressed the American people for the last time? At the beginning of his presidency, in 1981, I was at Harvard University. A gifted friend of mine from our schooldays, Jacek Hawiger, was then living and lecturing in Boston. Wishing to give me a pleasant evening after my lecture, he invited a group of Harvard luminaries to dinner. They included one Nobel Prize winner and several others who were obviously going to win Nobel Prizes. The dinner party went very well, until over dessert I admitted that it was time I congratulated them on their excellent president. The atmosphere soured instantly. First there was a silence, broken only by a few acid monosyllables, and then finally some perfunctory remarks were uttered, and the guests hurriedly dispersed. My words of rapture had ruined the whole dinner party. I know that even among sophisticated university intellectuals this attitude did gradually change to the president's benefit, and finally became established after his death. But over here in faraway Poland, we appreciated him from the start. For us he was the first president of a great country who was not afraid to call the "Evil Empire" by name and to throw down the gauntlet to it. That reminds me of New Year's Eve, 1983. In Poland martial law had been suspended, and over there, on the other side of the pond, preparations were already getting under way for the 1984 presidential election. We danced the night away at a forester's lodge near Gorc in the mountains, and in the morning we skied to first mass at a small wooden church in Niedźwiedź. The church was full to bursting. Lasses on the right, lads on the left, and the priest thundered away, presenting a vivid image of hell, with its gate standing open before us for last night's sinful, drunken debauch. The stench of hell fire filled the nave, and it felt as if the church, reeking of alcohol, would go up in one great flame. Finally the priest, *diminuendo* by now, said: "Once again I ask one thing of you. I've had enough trouble with this. Don't come to me after holy mass and don't leave me money to pray to the Lord God to beg for Reagan to be president again!"

How are we to cure the disintegration of memory, the characteristic feature of Alzheimer's disease, when we actually know so little about the memory? Since the 1970s more and more chemical molecules have been isolated that may play a role in the functioning of the memory, not just in us, but also in very different species such as snails, fruit flies and rodents. The implication is that the short-term memory, covering up to about twenty minutes, is based on chemical changes that strengthen existing connections (synapses) between nerve cells, while long-term memory, covering days and weeks, requires the production of new proteins and the creation of new connectors between the synapses. Recent research in animals indicates that ways of stimulating nerve cells that accompany learning new tasks are "acted out," repeated during sleep. So can it be that sleep consolidates and strengthens our memory? In the 1990s the dogma that said the nerve cells cannot regenerate and that we come into the world with a constant number of them was finally exploded. It turned out that of all the places in the brain, the hippocampus is "literally a breeding ground for nerve cells throughout life." Scientists have yet to determine to what degree these newly born cells support the working of the memory.

Can thoughts be sent? Transmitted at a distance? And with them emotions, desires and images? Not with the help of words, over the phone, by telegram or e-mail, but just by sheer will power, without the help of any gadgets or physical aids — directly from one brain to another, even if they are hundreds of miles apart. A young Prussian officer named Hans Berger believed in this mysterious form of communication after receiving a letter from his sister, in which she told him about a dream she had had in which he had fallen off his horse and been badly hurt. At just the same time he really had suffered the accident she described. After completing his military service, Berger — who was just starting out as a neurologist — devoted himself entirely to researching telepathy. He reckoned electromagnetic waves could be a vector for internal personal information. And in strict secrecy, in the basement of the hospital in Jena where he worked, for five years he measured and recorded the electrical currents in the brain, by means of electrodes attached to the skull. Although he was not the first person to conduct this sort of experiment, his observations were extremely precise and revelatory. He established that changes in the voltage, recorded by his string galvanometer, were not the outcome of fluctuations in blood pressure but arose in the cerebral cortex. However, the electrical field generated by millions of neurons proved to be thousands of times weaker than one created by an ordinary battery. This result must have disappointed the young experimenter. The electromagnetic waves emitted by one brain cannot be received by another brain; the voltage is too weak for them to move through the air. And although Berger never found proof for his concept of telepathy, he did make some fundamental observations that he published in 1928. He perceived the periodic nature of the rhythms of the brain, distinguishing alpha waves, beta waves and others, which science even wanted to name after him, though in his modesty he refused to give his consent. An example of rhythmical periodicity is sleep. Each of us goes through five successive phases during sleep, which show up separately on an electroencephalogram (EEG) recording; these phases are repeated several times a night, though their length varies from person to person. An EEG helps in diagnosing brain diseases, and allows us to observe the effect of drugs and sensory experiences. It also shows "the most striking, yet perhaps the least appreciated, behavior of the cortical networks is their regenerative, spontaneous activity" — throughout our lives.

In ascribing functions to individual areas of the brain some modern imaging techniques are helpful, such as positron emission tomography (PET), for example, and especially magnetic resonance imaging. This latter method enables us to measure the size of certain areas (morphometry), analyze their chemical composition (spectroscopy) and examine the flow of blood, as reflected in the consumption of oxygen or glucose by the brain (this is called functional magnetic resonance imaging). If in some area of the brain, usually one that is strictly defined, we observe features of an increased blood supply, small colored lights will appear on the monitor, and then we say that this region has been aroused and is working at full steam. And vice versa: impairment of these functions, for example in the hippocampus region, seems to be an early portent of Alzheimer's disease. The latest cameras have such high resolution that they can produce an image of perfect pitch! Or to put it a little more precisely, we can see the concentrations of cells in the cortex that are responsible for this unusual gift. Professional musicians have a better developed cerebellum (responsible for motor coordination) and occipital lobes, and they use Broca's center when they read, play or listen to music. Moreover, if we compare professional musicians with non-musicians, the former have more cerebral gray matter and lose less of it with the passage of time. So it is no surprise to hear that on learning of these results, a brilliant contemporary American neurologist declared: "Studying and performing music are good for the brain."

In a doctor's everyday work a musical education is not always particularly helpful. An ear for medicine does not go hand in hand with an ear for music. I have known experienced doctors who could not tell Bach and Stravinsky apart, but they could correctly diagnose a galloping heartbeat, which is very hard to hear, or a soft splitting of the second heart sound. However, I would be the last person to fail to appreciate the part played by music in medicine. Music shapes a doctor's sensitivity and awakens his sense of harmony and composition, whose instabilities find their reflection in illness.

By the third year of my studies I had forgotten about the brain, both the one on the kitchen table and the one under the skull. A friend and I used to drag ourselves off to the student science club at the Krakow Medical Academy's Pathological Anatomy Unit. There I attended dissections performed neatly and skillfully by Professor Janina Kowalczykowa. The clinician who was also required to be present was sometimes anxious and uncertain, because in those days the autopsy still counted as the final verification of a clinical diagnosis. Here, on the stage of the *theatrum anatomicum*, the professor calmly exposed to our view each of the organs in turn, probed their insides and found pathologies, while doing her best to show us as much as possible. In the late afternoon we would prepare histology specimens by cutting the organs into slivers, preserving them and dyeing them on microscope slides, with varying degrees of success and invariable reluctance — because we dreamed of doing our own autopsies. And just before the Christmas or Easter holidays, once the Unit had emptied and all the assistants had gone away, for half a pint of alcohol the lab technician — with the tacit consent of the head of the anatomy lab — would let us both into the room in the evening, where for hours on end we performed dissections. These were hours of solitary encounter with death, which tasted like a forbidden fruit. Totally absorbed, we used to make our way back down the long, dark corridors late at night, along avenues of display cases. On the shelves, crammed into jars, swimming in the depths of lemon-yellow formalin, were the most monstrous freaks of nature: little mermaids, cyclopses, cephalopods, limbless torsos, tumors baring a toothy grin and bulbous cancers. The formalin pathways were endless — we could feel ourselves growing fins, as on and on they carried us, until finally we saw the twinkle of streetlights and sighed with relief. A few days later the holidays were over, as were our adventures, and we were back to preparing slides. One day, in a second-hand bookshop I found a tattered French edition of *Recollections of My Life (Recollections de ma vie)* by Santiago Ramón y Cajal. The author's name meant nothing to me, but as I leafed through the book I realized he too had spent time making specimen slides. I bought the book for next to nothing, went home and could not tear myself away from it until dawn. That night I learned the story of one of the greatest discoverers of the brain.

Santiago Ramón y Cajal was born in 1852 on the slopes of the Pyrenees in a village whose fifty austere homesteads were hidden behind thick stone walls that had once protected the citizens against the Goths from the north and the Moors from the south. A stream flowed down from the mountains and cut across the marketplace. His father, the local doctor, devoted a lot of his time to educating the boy, and did so later on as well, when he and all four of his children had moved to a bigger place, Huesca, and then to Zaragoza. Apart from a love of drawing, which his father regarded as a waste of time, the boy showed no great distinction — except that he was interested in photography and making cannons. As leader of a small gang of boys his own age, he twice constructed a cannon that went off and blew up an iron garden gate, for which he went to prison for three days.

In 1877 he finished his medical studies and took a job in Valencia. He was consumed by a passion for research that attracted him to the invisible world revealed by the microscope. His laboratory was the domestic kitchen table. After supper, his plate was replaced by scientific instruments bought with his savings: a microscope, a simple implement for cutting organs into slivers (a microtome) made out of a barber's razor and about a dozen jars full of aniline and plant dyes. He would bring organs home from the mortuary or the abattoir, slice them up, dehydrate them in alcohol, immerse them in liquid paraffin, use the microtome to cut them into extremely thin slivers and stick them to microscope slides. Then he would dye them, mixing the colors, changing their temperature and exposure time, all in order to see the cells that same night. He would run out to the local café for a game of chess, go to bed for a short while, jump up before dawn and, using a fine pen and ink, draw what he had seen in the night under his microscope.

He grew more and more interested in the brain. In those days they already knew that it is made up of neurons — cells with a large number of radicular offshoots called dendrites, and one long, thin appendage, called the axon. For more than half the nineteenth century the argument went on simmering about the architecture of the brain and how exactly the branching neurons communicate with one another. It was generally believed that they were joined together by the appendages, that they were holding hands and interlacing, forming a tight network along which information flowed. However, there was no way of seeing this network. Applying the available techniques, scientists had dyed all the neurons and fibers without exception and seen a forest, but in its dense tangle the trees, leaves and roots were all lost from view. Then one of Cajal's contemporaries, an Italian named Camillo Golgi, made a breakthrough after years of laborious, persistent research. In difficult conditions, similar to those in which Cajal worked, he tested hundreds of dyes, varying their proportions, concentration and reaction time, in the belief that they would reveal to him the elusive structure. And finally he got it right: in scraps of brain steeped for some time in bichromate of potassium, and then in silver nitrate, the individual neurons showed. Their contours were bordered in a dark precipitate of silver. This reaction, in which the noble metal broke free, had something in common with alchemy. Even its name — Golgi called it a black reaction (*reazione nera*) — had an echo of *nigredo* ("blackening"), the first stage in which the alchemists used to carry out the "transmutation of forms that had been used up by Time."

Having become familiar with Golgi's technique, Santiago Ramón y Cajal hit upon the idea of using it to dye not the mature human brain, as other researchers were doing, but the brain of an embryo, where the network of neurons was far less dense. Once he had perfected the technique, he discovered that the nerve fibers (axons) end right next to the adjoining cell, but do not touch it. Between the axon and the cell it reaches, there is a narrow crack. And so the nervous system does not interlace to form a network, as Golgi ardently advocated. Instead, signals jump from cell to cell across a crack one twenty-millionth of a millimeter wide. This delicate, fragile connection, the substructure of neurobiology, is called the synapse. The transmission of signals in the synapse then turned out to be a complex process, involving the electrical depolarization of the cell membrane and the release of a wide variety of chemical transmitters. But how difficult it was to make a breakthrough with these revolutionary results! Cajal published them in Spanish, translated them into French himself and sent them to German periodicals, all without stirring any response. Then he realized that the world would only believe him when it saw the evidence with its own eyes. With the remains of his savings he bought a train ticket to Berlin and headed for the Anatomical Society Congress. There he set up his beloved microscope, borrowed several more, and displayed the specimen slides he had brought, such as no one had ever seen before. And it happened — he was finally noticed.

Meticulous, painstaking analysis of images under the microscope, recorded in the form of subtle, amazingly faithful drawings, enabled Cajal to define the route for the transmission of signals. They ran from inside a cell, down its long fiber to the neighboring cell, and their character was modulated by information flowing in earlier via hundreds of synapses. The numbers involved are enough to make your head spin. The human brain contains at least 10^{11} neurons; as on average a thousand synapses reach each one of them, the number of synapses is estimated at 10^{14}.

Cajal's discoveries led to the question of how stimuli are transmitted within the nervous system, provoking heated discussions that were still going on long after the scientist's death. It was reckoned that the nerves communicate with each other with the help of "sparks," or electrical currents. No one believed that chemical substances could provide an adequate speed of transmission. Nowadays, there is no doubt that inside the nerve transmission is electrical, but that at their endings the nerves secrete chemical compounds (neurotransmitters) that transfer impulses to other nerves or innervated cells. And so, for example, insufficient production in the synapses of the neurotransmitter called dopamine leads to Parkinson's disease. In 1906 the two great rivals, Santiago Ramón y Cajal and Camillo Golgi, jointly won the Nobel Prize. In their modest kitchen laboratories they had stared in solitude through the lenses of twin microscopes at the very same tissues, but each of them had seen a different nervous system. The scales had already tipped earlier in favor of Cajal, but to the end Golgi never abandoned faith in the correctness of his network theory. His Nobel lecture was one long venomous polemic attacking Cajal's views. The latter, meanwhile, a far more equable and good-natured person, had already said some years earlier: "What a cruel irony of fate to pair, like Siamese twins united by the shoulders, scientific adversaries of such contrasting characters!" But, nowadays, Golgi would have been pleased to see that in some areas of the brain, alongside the dominant synapses, nerve impulses can also be transmitted directly, from cell to cell, via protein channels linking them. And so the network over whose existence he fought a lifelong battle, though rudimentary, fragmented and local, does exist. Santiago Ramón y Cajal was not the only one who was right — a small bit of the truth was also due to Golgi!

How far do mental illnesses, known as illnesses of the soul, allow us to probe the depths of the brain? Psychiatry has always been torn between two visions of mental illness. One, based on the anatomy of the brain, its chemistry and pharmacology, associates mental disorders with the biology of the cerebral cortex. The other links the patients' afflictions with personal or social problems. In the history of psychiatry these two ways of looking, these two visions, have interwoven, and one or the other has taken precedence. When the foundations of psychiatry first began to emerge at some point in the eighteenth century, the biological concept prevailed. But the great intellectual trends of the nineteenth century brought "romantic psychiatry." Mental disorders began to be examined in terms of morality and passions. Passions were thought to arise spontaneously from the human soul. And in 1823 Johann Christian August Heinroth, director of the first university psychiatry faculty to be established in Germany, wrote: "Passions are like heated coals cast into the hotbed of life, or snakes oozing poison into the blood vessels, or vultures tearing at the entrails. As soon as it is ensnared by passion, the harmony of the individual is lost."

♦♦♦

The nineteenth century, especially its closing decades, through the mid-twentieth century was the era of lunatic asylums. The number of inmates grew at terrifying speed. Before the First World War, closed psychiatric hospitals had already become vast repositories, packed way beyond the limits of any chance of treatment, with the paralyzed, demented, feeble-minded and catatonic. They were places full of misfortune, petrified lives at a standstill, where all form of ties had been broken and the inmates suffered an endless death without dying. A closed hospital was a world apart, run according to its own set of rules, "a pitiful city full of perversions, made up of people no one needed, where time did not count, and where the only certainty was the lack of any prospect of a cure." The mental hospital was also compared to a giant monster "that sleeps all the time, without moving or dreaming; sometimes a risk of danger arose and then the monster awoke, grew anxious and filled everyone with fear, but then it fell asleep again." The "giant monsters" bursting at the seams only began to depopulate and lose their inmates in the 1960s and 1970s with the help of new drugs.

Among the inmates of closed lunatic asylums, a prominent place was occupied by patients suffering from progressive paralysis. As Tadeusz Boy-Żeleński wrote about them: "For progressive paralysis / Affects the noblest minds." This term defined cerebral syphilis. It manifested itself with psychopathological symptoms, and later dementia and paralysis. And in the words of Madame Marie Rivet, who ran a private hospital for the mentally ill in Paris in the 1870s, *la paralyse générale ne pardonne jamais* ("Progressive paralysis knows no mercy"). It was always fatal. In 1883 a young Austrian doctor named Julius Wagner-Jauregg noticed that in a syphilis patient who fell ill with erysipelas, the psychotic symptoms went into remission. Similar observations about the suppression of some illnesses by other, developing ones, have historically led to radical breakthroughs in therapy at least twice. And so it was this time too.

Wagner-Jauregg began to inject syphilis sufferers with tuberculin to induce a fever, and even achieved some lengthy remissions, though he stopped doing these experiments because of the presumed toxicity of tuberculin. In 1917 a thirty-seven-year-old actor was admitted to his hospital ward suffering from advanced neurosyphilis. He had profound memory dysfunction, convulsive fits and static pupils that failed to react to light, which meant the death sentence. Our doctor injected him with the blood of a soldier who had been brought back from the front in Macedonia suffering from malaria. Three weeks later the patient had his first attack of fever; after the tenth attack they started treating him with regular doses of quinine. In the months that followed his condition rapidly improved. From the vast repertoire in his memory he began to recite poetry and epic verse to an amazed audience, consisting of patients with skull injuries. Finally all the symptoms receded and he went back to work. It was an epoch-making moment in the history of psychiatry. For although "treatment by inducing fever" did not in fact lead to a complete cure, it changed the patients' fate so greatly that they did not die in a state of torpor, but could return to an almost normal way of life. This discovery, for which Wagner-Jauregg won the Nobel Prize, broke the barrier of therapeutic nihilism. It brought hope that if it was possible to arrest the progress of syphilitic psychoses, it might also be possible to stop psychoses of other origins.

Ultimately it was penicillin that dealt with syphilis, introduced into therapy in the 1940s. Meanwhile, neurotics were attracted by the phenomenal success of Freud's psychoanalytic theory, which dominated psychiatry for several decades, reaching its apogee in about the mid-twentieth century. For the first time psychiatrists began to receive patients at their own private consulting rooms for psychotherapeutic sessions. They filled the emotional gap in relations between doctor and patient, and created a cordial atmosphere, "in which the patients basked in what they believed to be an aura of concern." The enthusiasm of the middle class contributed to the success of psychiatry. Educated people were keen to discover more about themselves, to know the truth breaking through from the depths of the subconscious. Government agencies and the U.S. Congress turned to psychoanalysts with requests for consultations. Controlling neuroses seemed to be within reach. Freud and his pupils promoted the idea that they are derived from suppressed memories and sexual fantasies from childhood. A sophisticated procedure, including the analysis of dreams, free associations and renewed experience of neurosis-inducing situations from childhood made it possible to "work out diverse definitions of one's very self," and was supposed to bring liberation and recovery. Unexpectedly, however, in the 1970s rapidly growing cracks appeared in the mighty edifice of psychoanalysis, and the entire structure came tumbling down soon after. The leading experts on the subject who are its contemporaries say of psychoanalysis that it "was not a true methodology for treating psychological disturbances, but an opportunity to enhance one's personal growth and to engage in a self-indulging interior voyage." Others simply say that it was "an interruption, a hiatus" in the history of psychiatry. There are also those who go even further and claim that the fundamental ideas behind psychoanalysis are semantically empty concepts. As the renowned psychiatrist Hans Eysenck said in 1985: "All sciences have to pass through an ordeal by quackery.... Chemistry had to slough off the fetters of alchemy. The brain sciences had to disengage themselves from phrenology.... Psychology and psychiatry, too, will have to abandon the pseudo-science of psychoanalysis ... and undertake the arduous task of transforming their discipline into genuine science."

♦♦♦

Factors that have contributed to the decline of psychoanalysis in health care include the discovery of effective drugs, the establishment of a model for mental illnesses that places emphasis on neurogenesis, not psychogenesis, and the development of new methods of psychotherapy. The view that it was America and its great big pharmaceutical companies that killed psychoanalysis is not isolated — it died along with the generation of Jews who emigrated from Europe to escape racist persecution. Revolutionary changes in pharmacological treatment were the dominant factor, which began in the 1950s with the introduction of chloropromazine, and not long after benzodiazepines. At first attention was paid only to their suppressant effects; they were chemical straitjackets. Lunatics whose aggression was uncontrollable stopped shouting and became quiet. The new drugs gradually displaced traditional procedures such as electric shocks, insulin injections that put people into a state of lethargy or therapeutic showers, where they were struck on the head by alternate streams of very hot and ice-cold water. For the first time psychiatrists were starting to have strong sedating drugs at their disposal. Others followed, but in the 1990s Prozac took over. It went down a storm, becoming the tinderbox for a philosophy of pharmacological hedonism. Millions of completely healthy people began to demand a substance that would help them to bear the burden of existence . . . and keep a slender figure. Public acceptance of mental illnesses grew, and lunatics who had filled society with horror for millennia began to be regarded as people suffering from stress who could be helped. This change occurred not because we have become more understanding and tolerant, but because of Prozac — the prototype for a whole family of palliative drugs that calm mental illnesses.

This revolutionary — and indeed optimistic — breakthrough in therapy does not necessarily go hand in hand with understanding disorders in the functioning of the brain and the complexities of the human soul. Especially since in the case of neuroses, where what counts most of all is culture and social mores, biology does not have much to say. Whereas science itself, writes Edward Shorter, "wanders astray easily in the world of quotidian anxiety and sadness, in the obsessive traits of behavior and the misfiring personality types that are the lot of humankind." And, writing about the very faint dividing line between pathology and eccentricity, he concludes: "Despite its anchoring in the rest of medicine, psychiatry could easily drift aimlessly here." But what can be said about schizophrenics, into whose world we cannot find a way? What about unpredictable lunatics, who are especially dangerous in the persecution phase? If the patient thinks everyone else wants to kill him, it is highly likely that he will try to kill first as a means of self-defense. Such patients are "walking mines, just as dangerous to themselves as to others." It is because of them and others like them that impotence and doubt are always greater in psychiatry than in any other medical specialty. In answer to the question of how far we have come on the journey towards knowledge of the mind, the eminent contemporary expert on the subject Theodore Millon says: "A clear light does not appear to be in sight at the end of the tunnel; perhaps the field will never achieve anything close to a finite knowledge of mental reality." Despite this skepticism exuding pessimism, we should not forget that the image of mental illnesses has changed out of all recognition. Is it such a small thing that lunatics, or madmen, have been transformed into ordinary patients? For some of them, the combination of pharmacotherapy and psychotherapy has become an effective means of treating dysfunctions of the brain and mind.

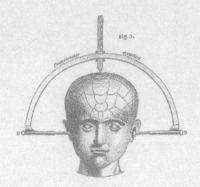

Fig 3.

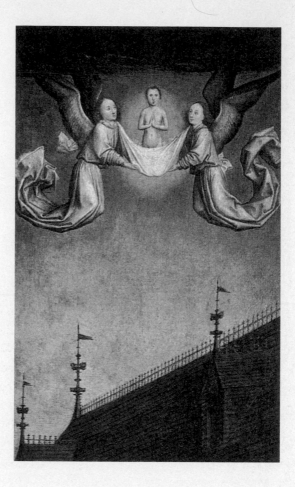

Simon Marmion
The Soul of Saint Bertin carried up to God, c. 1459
National Gallery, London

IN SEARCH OF THE SOUL

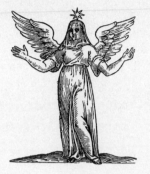

When we search for the origins of concepts, notions and ideas, we turn to the ancient Greeks. But where did they seek their sources? In Homer. They never looked further back; they were neither able to, nor did they believe it necessary. The heroes of *The Iliad* and *The Odyssey* viewed the world without illusions and faced up to its challenges without feeling sorry for themselves. To them the human condition was final. Ananke and her laws hung inevitably overhead, the course of life was already marked out and there was no way to change it in any circumstances. So they knew life without salvation, without rescue, without any hope of it recurring; "it is only because life is irretrievable ... that the glory of appearance can reach such intensity." And that is why Achilles says:

> Cattle and sheep are things to be had for the lifting,
> and tripods can be won and the tawny high heads of horses,
> but a man's life cannot come back again, it cannot be lifted
> nor captured again by force, once it has crossed the teeth's
>   barrier.

These lines, referring to the transience of life, its non-recurrence, have been much admired. They have lost none of their force over the centuries. Thus nowadays too, "whenever somebody who doesn't belong to any creed refuses to kill, Achilles's words live on in him." But what about the soul? It flew away to the underground kingdom of the shades, from which there was no return. So when Odysseus goes to see Achilles in Hades, he tries to comfort him and lavishes words of admiration on him, saying that even in the underworld he "has preserved his 'great power,'" but Achilles replies:

> *O shining Odysseus, never try to console me for dying,*
> *I would rather follow the plow as a thrall to another*
> *man, one with no land allotted to him and not much to*
> > *live on,*
> *than be a king over all the perished dead . . .*

The Greeks of the Homeric era were not the first or the only people to wonder about man's fate after his demise. Almost all human tribes have asked themselves, at an early point in their history, whether man's conscious personality can survive after death. Almost all have answered in the affirmative. "On this point, sceptical or agnostic peoples are nearly, if not wholly unknown," said the famous ethnologist J.G. Frazer. From the household items found in tombs we know that as early as the Neolithic era the citizens of the Aegean region felt that the human need for food, drink, clothing and even entertainment did not stop with death. There is no evidence to prove that some sort of theories about life beyond the grave lay hidden behind this practice. In the Balkans the custom of feeding the dead through tubes, which was just as widespread as in archaic Greece, survived almost to the present day.

✦✦✦

Homer uses two words to refer to the soul. Usually it is the *thymós*, which can be broadly defined as the seat of the emotions. Whereas he seems to ascribe the word *psyché* to man at the moment of his death, in his agony, when he is profoundly unconscious or his life is in danger. And so the only stated function of the *psyché* is to leave the body when life is extinguished. So what else do we know about the *psyché*? It features as a character in an ancient myth that has survived to this day in the Latin version by Apuleius. In it, Psyche appears as a very lovely young Sicilian princess, of immense, enchanting beauty. Enraged by her loveliness, the furious Aphrodite sends Eros to punish her, but he falls madly in love with her instead. He carries her off to a wonderful palace in a flowery valley shielded by rocky crags and visits her by night. But he warns her never to try to find out who he is, because the sight of his face will be the beginning of her days of misery. Her sisters decide he must be a monster, a beast, as he will not let her look at him. Unable to conquer her curiosity, one night as Eros is sleeping, Psyche approaches him with an oil lamp. Dazzled by his unearthly beauty, she shudders and a drop of hot oil falls on his divine shoulder. The miracle vanishes, Eros disappears along with the fairytale palace, and the princess is left alone among the wild rocks. She roams the Earth, rejected by all, until Aphrodite catches her, imprisons her in her palace and sets her work beyond her strength. She takes vengeance on Psyche, "causing pain, distress and torment," but Eros, who has not stopped loving her, brings her help and consolation. Finally Zeus takes pity on the lovers. He receives Psyche on Olympus, grants her immortality and celebrates her marriage to the god of love. And so Psyche had the features of the human soul: she was beautiful, curious and disobedient to a god. However, her difficult earthly wanderings came to an end in heaven, where love had taken her.

◆◆◆

In the post-Homeric era the word *psyché* appears on the lips of the Greeks more and more often. It is the mental counterpart of the body, and at first it is not in conflict with it. It dwells somewhere in the depths of the organism, and from these inner parts it is able to address its owner in its own voice. In about the fifth century BC the meaning of the word *psyché* reaches a turning point and changes completely. Now man is endowed with a hidden "self" of divine significance. The body and the soul are now at two opposite poles. Through purification, the soul can liberate itself from the body and — as Pythagoras taught — be reborn in a new body. This was an absolute novelty, unknown to Homer's heroes, an astonishing interpretation of life, a concept that has been defined as "a drop of alien blood in the veins of the Greeks." Scholars have combed the horizon in search of the source from which this drop could have fallen. Many have looked towards Asia Minor and beyond, focusing their suspicions on the shamans. In the seventh century BC, when the Black Sea region opened to Greek colonization — writes the eminent expert on the ancient world, E.R. Dodds — the Greeks came into contact with shaman culture. So it may have been from the shamans that they got inspiration for new ideas about the soul that were alien to Achilles and his comrades. By this route some very powerful stimuli reached them that may have engendered the Pythagorean mysteries and enabled Plato to discover a world of ideas that one day, centuries later, would open up the afterworld: heaven, purgatory and hell.

Shaman culture still exists in Siberia, among the Yakuts, and evidence of its existence in the remote past has been left over a vast area, stretching from Scandinavia right across the land mass of Eurasia, all the way to Indonesia. We are aware of it largely thanks to the Polish exiles who were sent to Siberia. As early as 1768 the tsar ordered ten thousand of the Bar Confederates — nobles who tried to defend Polish independence — to be conscripted into the most distant garrisons on the frontiers of Siberia. The writings from Siberia of Bronisław Piłsudski, brother of the Marshal, or of Wacław Sieroszewski are real treasure-troves of information on the shamans, and to this day their observations are being continued by ethnologists based in Poznań. The world outlook of the shamans differs from the world view of sorcerers, magicians and enchanters, who can still be found in some places on Earth today. They all tried, or still try, to drive evil spirits out of the sick. But only the shaman followed the sick to a place where no one else even imagined it was possible to go.

At dusk, after separating the yurt housing the sick man from the rest of the universe by ramming poles into its outside with birds' and horses' heads stuck on top and tying young birches together with ropes made of horse hair, the shaman would drive away accidental spirits and summon good ones to his aid. Then, in a growing state of ecstasy and *kamlanie*, he would begin his negotiations with the spirits of disease for the soul of the sick man. Here is how Wacław Sieroszewski describes the shamanic ritual of *kamlanie*: "Total, agonizing silence—until suddenly, from God knows where, a harsh, fitful screech rings out, as piercing as the rasp of metal . . . and falls silent. Later again . . . , a seagull cries pitifully, a falcon shrieks, and a curlew whistles . . . It was the shaman screaming, modulating his voice; and then silence again, just a very faint trembling, like the buzz of a mosquito, shows that the sorcerer has started his music. The drum beat . . . increases, grows stronger, pauses, and once again . . . breaks off. To the capricious thud of the drum, the wildest sounds fly past in zigzags: eagles cry, seagulls complain, black loons snigger, curlews squeal, and cuckoos cuckoo. As if all those flying near heaven had suddenly stopped, surrounded the sorcerer in a swarm and were accompanying him, warning the occupants of heaven of his march with their pitiful cry." Amid this music, in a profound state of ecstasy, having negotiated the rate of the sacrifice, the shaman did something highly original, unknown to any other healers and magicians: he followed the soul of the sick man into "the other world." He raised himself to each of its successive levels, making an offering at each one, until finally he reached the right spot, where he exchanged the sacrifice for the soul of the sick man. He placed it in his ear and went back to Earth; his return manifested itself as an unconscious state of prostration into which he fell. As soon as he recovered consciousness, he would blow the soul into the crown of the patient's head, or beat it into him with a stick.

We can find evidence of the shamans in the myth of Orpheus. He is a combination of a poet, a magician and a prophet. Like the legendary shamans of Siberia, he can control bird music and wild animals. Just like shamans worldwide, he visits the afterworld to recover a stolen soul. Finally, as a magic "self," he goes on living in the form of a singing head that remains an oracle many years after his death. The myth of Orpheus was the inspiration for an entire cult, whose adherents believed that—like Orpheus—they would find the way from the world above to the underworld, and would manage to cheat death. In the Orphic mysteries they cut themselves off increasingly from the world of the senses, developing ideas about being cleansed of sin and about life beyond the grave. If, moreover, we remember that Orpheus's motherland was Thrace, where the Greeks had their earliest contact with shaman culture, we are not surprised by Professor Dodds's potent claim that Orpheus is a Thracian, mythical shaman or the prototype for a shaman. This myth about a man who sets off alone into the afterworld to recover the soul of a sick person makes a beautiful backdrop for medicine. Just like the mystery of *katharsis*. We can imagine that in ancient times, Greek genius made an unusual shift in concepts, "replacing" shamanism with *katharsis*. Both are accompanied by psychological shock. But in order to restore health, to release someone from illness, you no longer have to break free of the body and fly into the unexplored world beyond. It is enough to free the body from evil, to purify it. If evil is located in the soul, art will bring *katharsis*, and if in a sickness of the body, medicine will bring it.

In the soul, our dream of immortality is reflected, as in a mirror. For this dream to come true, we would only have to revoke the irreversibility of time. In contemplating nature, the Greeks became convinced that it was possible, and that it did in fact happen. They saw the regular motion of the stars, the invariable cycle of days and nights, births and deaths, and animals behaving in the same way. In the eyes of those who had been observing nature for centuries it seemed to exist without time, "or at least to lack irreversible time." It seemed unaware of a past that was lost and gone once and for all. This perspective shaped itself into the concept of eternal recurrence: the world is constantly returning to where it began, though great abysses of time separate these returns. Because the world has a finite number of particles, and thus also a finite number of systems, hence every system must recur an infinite number of times. This concept "took hold in European thought with astonishing staying power." It appeared in the works of Plato, Epicurus and the Stoics, to survive for centuries and turn up in the work of Schopenhauer, who wrote: "We can compare time to an endlessly revolving sphere; the half that is always sinking would be the past, and the half that is always rising would be the future." The highest point of the wheel was supposed to be the present, motionless, and always the same. A thoroughly original attempt to understand the contradictory, mutually exclusive concepts of eternity and transience was undertaken by Friedrich Nietzsche. And after ten years of thought, out of the mountains, down to the people he sent Zarathustra, the advocate of eternal recurrence.

The theory, or rather fantasy of eternal recurrence is a comforting idea. These days, however, it does not have many adherents, and in the Christian tradition it met with determined opposition, from Saint Augustine, for example. So if not in eternal recurrence, where should we seek the fulfillment of the eternal dream that something more of us than just dust will remain? Something that never dies, that is stronger than death and that lasts forever. Like words enclosed in a hexameter, more enduring than bronze: "I shall not altogether die." A strong conviction, repeated centuries later, in defiance of "desolate times": "But that which endures the poets give." They are the select few "who knew the secret of word spells, time-resistant forms without which ... speech is like sand." What else might remain? The laws of nature, the great theorems of mathematics? And love. Because "the value of human life is measured above all by love. Love also determines a man's saintliness to a fundamental degree." That was said by the man at the news of whose death hundreds of thousands of people cried out: *Santo subito!* The rest of us try to find an anchorage (however slight the chances of success), a permanent element in what is granted us, what is closest to us:

> *And if indeed you should silently utter*
> *the same old words you always hide and burn,*
> *you won't leave a footstep behind you, little man,*
> *but a point of light, the glimmer of a glowworm.*

Where in our bodies was this personification of immortality supposed to be located? The Egyptians pointed to the heart, but the Greeks placed the soul elsewhere. They imagined it "in the form of a little doll, visible through the pupil of the eye, which as a result they called the *kore*." In Greek *kore* means little girl, or doll, and also the pupil of the eye. How did the Greeks know that the pupil is the only natural window with a view of the brain, of its optic nerves? The image of a little girl has been permanently associated with the pupil of the eye ever since doctors started calling it the *pupilla*, which is the Latin for "little girl."

Who first uttered the word *kore*? Was it a father gazing at his daughter? Or a boy looking at his girlfriend? Or maybe it was a child, because there are words that may have fallen from the lips of children before entering the adult dictionary and taking up permanent residence there. That was apparently the case with the Latin equivalent of *kore*. The word *pupa* and its diminutive, *pupilla*, meaning a little girl or a doll, were first heard in the prattle of Roman toddlers. The same is true of *papa* as a name for a father. But in the case of *kore* there is no such conjecture. The word is very old, lost in the mists of time. It was on the lips of the Achaeans, and it was taken over by their conquerors, the Dorians. It appears very often in Homer. In pre-Homeric times it had not yet crystallized in a single form and was pronounced in several different ways. In its oldest form it took the phoneme "v" in the middle and sounded like *kuor.v.e.* The differences gradually faded out and the only versions to last were *kore* (κόρη) in the Attic dialect, *kure* (κώυρη) in the Ionian dialect and *kora* (κώρα) in the Doric.

Only once did *kore* substitute for a proper name. It was given to a beauty without a name, the daughter of Zeus and Demeter. She was so admired and desired on Olympus for her loveliness that her mother decided it would be safer to move her to Earth. In central Sicily to this day they will show you the meadow where Kore and a group of other girls used to play and pick flowers. This sort of scene had irresistible charm for the gods; we only have to think of the rape of Europa, among others. This time the Earth opened, and out onto its surface drove a golden chariot harnessed to a team of four black horses. Hades, ruler of the underworld, had come to kidnap Kore—who from then on bore the gloomy name Persephone—and make her queen at his side. Just before he arrived, a beautiful narcissus had bloomed in the meadow. Kore was gazing at the narcissus, which was also the name of the youth who became lost as a result of gazing at himself. Perhaps she thought she had found the ultimate vision. She stretched out her hand to seize it, but at that moment Hades emerged. A scream rang out. Was it just the scream of the kidnapped girl? Or also the scream of irreversible knowledge? Kore saw herself, double, reflected in the eye of Hades, whose name means "invisible." From then on she was to become the pupil of the eye—and that was to apply to all of us. There she remained, in the eye that "pounced from the shadows to capture a girl and shut her away in the underworld palace of the mind."

The rest of the story is well known. Demeter—the *mater dolorosa* of antiquity—wandered the world in a ragged dress, with her hair loose and scattered in ashes, searching for her daughter everywhere, but in vain. Then this goddess of the harvest, the patroness of farmers, caused a drought on Earth. Zeus gave way and ordered Hades to set Persephone free. In parting, he gave her a pomegranate, and she ate a few grains, not knowing that just this tiny morsel would tie her forever to the kingdom of the shades. From then on, every year, she had to return to the Underworld for six months. When she emerged in spring, the world decked itself in flowers, so great was the joy of Demeter, who had not forgotten her. And so they were parted and reunited, becoming more and more of a single being in two persons. It was a "drama of the reflection," breaking free of the body, the Earth, and then recombining with its point of departure. It was a profound mystery. And for centuries the Greeks worshipped the reflected image, as in the pupil of the eye, that pervaded the entire enigma, in their most arcane Eleusinian Mysteries, celebrated for the twofold goddess, Demeter-Kore.

In Greek or Roman written sources, including medical texts, it is not easy to find a precise description of the view, cited by Jan Parandowski, among others, that "the little doll" appearing in the pupil of the eye is the soul personified. Relatively closest to this concept are an extract from a discourse in Pliny the Elder's *Naturalis Historia* and a passage from Pseudo-Plato's *Alcibiades*. Pliny draws attention to the small dimensions of the pupil, which "do not permit the sight to wander at hazard and with uncertainty, but direct it as straight as though it were through a tube," and a little further on he enthuses that "so complete a mirror, too, does the eye form, that the pupil, small as it is, is able to reflect the entire image of a man." And as Socrates says to Alcibiades, the pupil is the part of the eye "that is noblest." And if, as Socrates would have it, the Delphic maxim "Know thyself" can only be understood when it is translated into "Look at thyself," in this understanding "the eye became the pupil for us all." And the eye, if it "is to see itself, must look at an eye," and "if the soul is to know herself, she must surely look at a soul, and especially at that region of it in which occurs the virtue of a soul."

At the moment of death the soul was liberated from the cocoon of the body and flew away like a butterfly into the afterworld. This is how we see it on Greek cameos with portraits of the dead and on Roman sarcophagi. In Greek the word *psyché* also means a butterfly, to which Aristotle drew attention, and in Latin the word *anima* can be used to mean either the soul, or a moth or butterfly. Juliusz Słowacki saw the soul as a swallow taking flight from the eye at the onset of death, and prayed for intercession for it in these lines:

> *Or rather I shall say — as the dusk of this life draws nigh*
> *The soul is like a swallow high above the Earth,*
> *Succor the swallow as it flies from my eye*
> *Gaze to the sunlight, heart full of mirth.*

But doesn't the soul "take flight" every night? Doesn't it soar as the body sleeps? Doesn't it liberate itself from the body, take off and break free? So is sleep, by setting the soul free, a paraphrase of death? The Greeks noticed this affinity. To them, Hypnos, the god of sleep, and Thanatos, the god of death, were twins, the sons of the Night. They imagined Hypnos as a winged youth who touches the brows of the weary with a twig, or scatters poppyseed on them from a corner. Whereas they saw Thanatos as a boy holding the torch of life, extinguished and turned upside down. They were attached to each other as only twins can be. According to Jan Kochanowski, Hypnos, the mirror image of Thanatos, heralded his coming:

> O sleep, that teaches all people to die
> And shows them the taste of the future life

The god of sleep had power over man, cutting down the victors and making no exceptions, not even for the noblemen of Dobrzyń, as Adam Mickiewicz jokingly testified in *Pan Tadeusz*:

> On tankard, plate and sirloin in a heap,
> The victors vanquished by Death's brother, Sleep.

If the soul is liberated from the body during sleep, through how many worlds does it wander, worlds that exist for a moment, before being forgotten forever? And would we like someone very dear to us to accompany us in these dream worlds, to be with us in a place where the real world no longer burdens us, where we sense the only opportunity to be fully united:

> Take me into your dream
> Let me stay within it

Let me revolve inside it
until I melt entirely
underneath your eyelids.

Sleep also brings fears, or even terror. For me it was the return of my stage fright. The dream came to me long after I had stopped performing music in public and taken up medicine "for real." It used to wake me up, terrified, covered in sweat. In the dream I came out on stage and sat at the piano, and then the auditorium went quiet, but I couldn't remember the first note. In my short and far from successful musical career, this never actually happened. Of course, I made mistakes, I fluffed—as we used to say at school—on more than one occasion I bungled whole passages, but as for not being able to start at all, that never happened to me! Nor to any of the musicians I have known. Indeed, years later, when I mentioned this dream to the brilliant pianist Janusz Olejniczak, winner of the Chopin competition, he replied: "Do you know, I have exactly the same dream! I come out on stage and sit down at the piano, and then I notice I've got the wrong notes, a different score. I am unable to begin, and I wake up covered in sweat." So I felt less alone with the stage fright that was torturing me in my sleep after all those years.

The god of sleep flew right around the world with the onset of night. How did he know its limits? "When does the night end and the day begin?" the tzaddik asked a large gathering of Hasidic Jews. And gave the answer himself: "When in the eyes of another man you see a brother."

Heraclitus ascribed the role of the world's first principle to the soul. He believed that one of its features was the *lógos*, which surpassed it and was identical with the Logos of the universe. The Logos is reason, the cosmic force, the divine law that unites all changeable objects and rules over them. In modern times Imre Kertész referred to it in talking about the written word: "*Logos*, the invisible spider's thread that holds our lives together" and ceaselessly goes on creating it. Heraclitus warned: "Of the soul thou shalt never find boundaries, not if thou trackest it on every path," and in a footnote he specified: "so deep is its *lógos*." Does that mean searching for the soul is doomed to failure from the outset? Is it like hunting the Snark? An expedition in search of the Yeti? Aiming to achieve the impossible?

The Siberian shamans had not read Heraclitus when they devised their methods of reaching the soul. The training took years on end. The pupil, carefully selected by the teacher, began living in isolation, performing painful, repulsive and shattering exercises in order to kill the instinct to run away from anything dangerous and terrifying. Extreme exhaustion led to the collapse of his former personality, because "the shaman must die in order to be born anew." The central experience of this initiation was the disintegration of the body. So, for example, among the Eskimos a monstrous polar bear would devour the apprentice's body in a dream, leaving nothing but bones "that then grew a new body around them." And finally, after many years, once the pupil had conquered his own "initiation sickness" and cured himself of it, only then could he practice the art he had acquired on others. He was capable of seeing through matter and catching sight of the spirit that filled it. He could not only see "the other world," but he could communicate with it. No one was as good as the shaman, "a seasoned expert on the topography of the afterworld," at tracking a lost or abducted soul and battling with its kidnappers to regain it for the sick person. He did it in the state of ecstasy that he had learned during the long initiation process. There was a wide range of psychotropic drugs to help him, including hallucinogens, such as extracts of fly agaric or bog bilberry, and especially certain varieties of bracket fungus. So too, three thousand years before Christ, the stimulating fruit bodies of a species of bracket fungus called *Piptoporus betulinus* (the birch bracket) were threaded on a piece of string and taken with him on his journey by Ötzi, the man whose frozen remains were found not long ago in an Alpine glacier. He hadn't had time to use them before his soul flew from his body.

The shamans came close to the essential experience that seizes a man when he is in a state of ecstasy. In these exceptional, privileged moments they tried to go beyond the apparent and accessible world, and to penetrate the hidden one, to tear down the curtain concealing all that is most essential. Plotinus knew about this, and referred to ecstasy, the height of rapture, a revelation, as the only way of merging with the absolute. It was not just a cognitive function, and "demanded not studying, but exercising the spirit (*askesis*) and purification (*katharsis*)." For Plotinus had no doubt that there really was an existence more perfect than Plato's ideas — the height of beauty, truth, goodness and unity — the absolute, or "The One" (τὸ ἕν). Divine existence, we would say. The human "self," hidden in the soul, is not inseparably divided from the eternal "self" present in the divine mind. This real "self," the "self" within God, is also granted to me within me. And when the internal pressure intensifies, Plotinus taught, until ecstasy comes upon us, we identify with it, we become identical with it, its ineffable beauty raises us up and we are united with the divine thought that contains us. Then we experience an overwhelming sensation of peace, joy, happiness and contact with the ultimate meaning. And everything around us takes on unutterable beauty and perfection, and turns out exactly as it should be.

Seventeen centuries separate us from Plotinus. History has

carried us a long way from the wise man who died alone at his villa in Campania. Yet if we read the pages of his *Enneads* today, they still stir an echo in us. Henri Bergson wrote about this power to influence that the mystics have: "They ask nothing, and yet they receive. They have no need to exhort; their mere existence suffices." By existing, they challenge us. Plotinus knew well that a man's inner life will never be made whole: "it will never be pure ecstasy or pure reason or pure animality." He encourages us to be open to transcendence. In the rare moments of inspiration and elation that he called "the escape of the recluse to the Recluse," the soul of Plotinus turned to it, the One and Only that created our world. "Let then every man become divine and every man beautiful, if he wants to see God and beauty," he wrote. "We are given the impression that this imperative of his is somehow connected by invisible threads with the ultimate mystery of the universe," said Lev Shestov. Plotinus was to experience four ecstasies. After the first one he wanted nothing but to be in anticipation of the one and only voice. Perhaps this was comparable to the state we sometimes experience when listening to a rondo. The first time it appears, it is a dazzling theme. After a while it vanishes, leaving us enthralled. Now we are just waiting, with all our hearts and minds, for its return.

Mystical experience is a universal phenomenon. "Even if this phenomenon attains its plenitude only with Christianity, it nevertheless exists, in a highly authentic way, throughout human history. The Plotinian experience is one of the most remarkable examples of this." He was one of the first in a long line of great mystics who described their revelations, including the following saints: John of the Cross, Hildegard of Bingen, Catherine of Siena and Teresa of Ávila. They all presented us with their "most vital experience, which tells the truth about oneself and the world, and has its origin in the depths of the human soul." And the great female ecstatics! Whether in a state of rapture or in the depths of suffering, immersed in revelation, between ardor and the throes of death, mad, and yet fulfilled—for centuries they have not ceased to feed the imagination of painters and sculptors, "often less pious than their heroines." *The Ecstasy of Saint Teresa*, sculpted by Bernini, can be seen in a chapel in a small church in Rome, Santa Maria della Vittoria. The chapel is built in the shape of a theater, with an audience consisting of the figures of the donors, sitting in the boxes, watching the scene being acted out before them, and which was described by the saint herself. Teresa is resting on a cloud; her mouth is part open and her eyes are half closed. Above her, with a slight smile that may be tender or cruel, depending from what angle you look at it, or perhaps simply mischievous, stands a very young angel holding up an arrow that he is just about to stab into her heart. He seems to be enjoying the saint's state of ecstasy. Yet above all it is the face of Saint Teresa that has attracted our gaze for centuries—the face of a woman in elation, a woman anticipating, desiring, a woman in a state of celestial bliss.

An account of the revelation experienced by Blaise Pascal has also survived to our times. He was thirty-one years old; it was Monday, 23 November 1654, in Paris. The time: between ten-thirty PM and half past midnight. That night he saw a great light and a blinding fire. For a long time he passed out, and as soon as he regained consciousness, he immediately wrote down his experiences with a steady hand, on paper. As he had a scientific mind, he began by stating the time and the place, as quoted above. Further on, after an address to the biblical God of the Old Testament, the style becomes telegraphic. Repeated several times over, the word "certainty" is striking, and so are "joy" and "peace." And a desire to forget about everything except God. He carried the note he had written in a state of revelation to the end of his life, sewn into the lining of his jacket. He was accused on more than one occasion of fundamentalism (a pejorative word in the era of globalization); of making a mockery of reason, which in fact he used to make some brilliant discoveries in mathematics and physics; of ruthlessness and of stripping everything bare. But he never forgot the moment that raised his soul and changed the world, and never let it slip into oblivion. Mad? Of course—in the sense of being different, of rejecting the world, which from then on ceased to exist for him. All that counted was the love he had experienced in his revelation.

Pascal had more luck with witches than with doctors. His sister Gilberte said he never knew a day without pain and suffering. In the first year of his life he was already racked with convulsions. The doctors were helpless, and finally his desperate father, who adored him all his life, thought he must be under a spell cast by an old hag whom his wife had refused a handout. Under the threat of the stake, the old woman admitted it. She offered to transfer the charm from the child to a black cat. She made a potion and prayed to Satan. The cat expired, but the child did not get better. Then, aware that the stake was getting closer, she made "a cataplasm of nine leaves from three different plants that were picked during a full moon by a seven-year-old child." When she applied this cataplasm, the little boy was shaken with a terrible fit of convulsions, and sank into a state of catalepsy. The frantic father went for the witch with his fists flying. Just then the child awoke from his coma and smiled. The witch announced that he was cured. The attack abated, never to return.

Many times in youth and adulthood, Pascal was chained to his bed by migraines and stomach pains. So it was in September 1647, when Descartes, on his way back from Sweden, stopped in Paris for three days before moving to Amsterdam for good. He had heard a lot about the young genius, so he invited him to come to see him. Pascal replied that he was feeling too unwell to go to the other end of Paris, which Descartes regarded as impertinence on his part. However, he would not wait, so the day before his departure he—the greatest philosopher in Europe—decided to go to see the young man of twenty-four. He found him in bed, and asked him detailed questions about the symptoms, not just to assure himself that his host really was ill, but also because he regarded himself as a medical man. Pascal did not give a single word in reply because he did not like to complain in front of strangers. Later on, he showed Descartes his arithmetic machine—the prototype of the modern computer—and some tubes for creating a vacuum. Descartes was so fascinated by the brilliant young man that the next day, before leaving, he visited him once again.

Both of these great mathematicians, by way of skepticism, attained diametrically different philosophical positions. Pascal reached mysticism, with an infinite predominance of the soul over the body, the soul in which the preternatural order is reflected in love. It was said of him that "never was philosophy deeper felt; it was not the result of a mighty inner struggle," and so for all time he found people for whom he was a guide. Descartes, like no one before him, radically divided the world of thought from the material world, the soul from the body. He believed that these two separate worlds communicate with each other in the pineal gland, a tiny anatomical growth situated at the base of the brain, where the soul was supposed to reside. The pineal gland is a third eye. In bony fish, the oldest amphibians and the first reptiles, it remained in the forehead, enabling them to look upwards, and has been preserved in fossils. It exists to this day as a third eye in just one reptile, the tuatara, a spiny lizard-like creature that lives on an island off the New Zealand coast. In all other ancestral species it disappeared in the Triassic period and gradually became hidden deep in the brain. It has preserved its connection with the visual system, and especially at night it produces melatonin, a hormone that is involved in measuring out the rhythm of sleep and waking, and is also used nowadays to prevent jet lag after transoceanic flights. Descartes could not have known the pineal gland was the remnant of a third eye, and yet, like the Greeks, he located the soul in the eye, this time the third one!

Descartes was a dualist, and defended Christian views from increasing materialism. But the further development of human thought headed in this very direction. The philosophers of the Enlightenment and their successors smashed the dualist concept that Descartes had artificially concocted with the help of the pineal gland, and started explaining all spiritual matters as material phenomena. In the sphere of philosophy the old order was reversed: philosophy became a science of pure thinking, only concerning itself with existences in so far as they are present within our consciousness, and not just insofar as they exist outside us. The whole great drama of the history of redemption disappeared in the Enlightenment mentality. As John Paul II wrote: "According to the logic of *cogito, ergo sum* God was reduced to an element within human consciousness; no longer could he be considered the ultimate explanation of the human *sum*. Nor ... the one who gives existence.... All that remained was the idea of God, a topic for free exploration by human thought."

How can we see the soul, if only for a moment? Where should we look for it? Lie in wait for it as it leaves the body? After all, Achilles spoke of that moment, and Słowacki wrote about it. The curiosity of Frederick II, son of King Roger, the hero of Karol Szymanowski's opera, was legendary. We do not know if he based his plans on Achilles's words; certainly not on Słowacki's. This powerful ruler of the Norman state of Sicily reportedly gave orders for a man to be shut in a barrel and starved to death, because he wanted to see the soul departing. History is silent on whether or not he succeeded. After the Enlightenment the issue seemed simpler. Indeed, matter turned out to be all, and everything was made of it, including the soul. And so the soul must have a mass; it must be subject to the laws of gravity and be possible to weigh. So reasoned Duncan MacDougall in 1901, a doctor at the city hospital in Haverhill, Massachusetts. As a man of action he soon stopped philosophizing and got down to work. He used a crane scale, on which he placed a bed with a dying man in it. For four hours he took meticulous measurements. He observed the patient carefully until the man emitted his last breath. And at that moment the beam of the scale dropped; the body had lost weight! He repeated his experiment four more times—always with the same result. However, when dogs were used instead of people, the result was unambiguously negative. Only people, but not dogs, suddenly lost weight at the moment of decease. If it was the soul flying from the body, then it "weighed as much as a slice of bread." MacDougall kept the results of his observations secret, but as rumors of his astounding research spread, he was finally prompted to publish in a medical journal a work entitled *The Soul: Hypothesis Concerning Soul Substance Together with Experimental Evidence of the Existence of Such Substance.* Despite this rather pompous title, the work is striking for the precision of his observations, his solicitous control of the conditions for the experiments, and his cautious reasoning. Some say that even today it should be put through the rigorous filter of the review process and see the light of day again. An independent confirmation of the results would be expected, of course. To which MacDougall would surely have referred to the results of observations made by a Californian high school teacher, who thirty years later conducted an analogous experiment on mice. As they expired, the unfortunate mice did not lose weight. Ah, but they were mice, not people. He would also surely have referred to recently mooted suggestions that convection currents could provide a partial explanation for his insights. To the ultimate accusation of exuberant originality, MacDougall could have said that five thousand years before him the ancient Egyptians wrote about weighing the soul, which was located in the heart, after death. To be pure, a heart tossed on the scales at a posthumous trial before Osiris had to weigh less than the lightest feather. "Otherwise, it was immediately gobbled up by a monster waiting by, and the Egyptian's life beyond the grave ended in eternal ignominy."

Reducing the soul to a material substance and trying to capture it on a scale are derivatives of the Cartesian doubt that has accompanied us for the past four hundred years. For many long centuries before then, the world was full of evidence of God. God was nearby and present within our souls, where He manifested Himself simply as the truth. And so Saint Augustine could say: "Do not come out into the world, return to yourself, the truth lives inside a man." And he added: "I desire to know God and the soul. Nothing more? Absolutely nothing." After Descartes there was only the God of rational religion, the God of people of the Enlightenment, "a high-ranking officer in the moral police," who deserved nothing else "except the *coup de grâce* that Feuerbach, Nietzsche and Freud later delivered him." Human reason had emancipated itself and ceased to need — so they said — this crutch, this working hypothesis. The nihilism that Nietzsche was the first to perceive on the threshold of Europe entered by the front door. Right at the end came the Marxist utopia, the ultimate version of the Enlightenment belief in progress and heaven on earth, prepared by the powers of reason. Confidence in the meaning of the whole of reality was deeply disturbed, and the world became more and more empty and difficult to understand. The French thinker Pierre Delalande, invented by Vladimir Nabokov in the novel *The Gift*, says: "In our earthly house, windows are replaced by mirrors." This means we are incapable of looking outside worldly life to see what is in the world beyond. It also means we can only see ourselves.

Even assuming that is the truth, a great deal depends on what sort of look we aim at the mirror. As in the story about the dog that runs into a series of rooms with walls entirely covered in mirrors. The only door slams shut behind him, and there he stands, surrounded on all sides by dogs—his own reflection in the mirrors. He bares his fangs, and so do they. He flies at them, and they fly to him. Faster and faster he races, louder and louder he barks, foaming more and more fiercely at the mouth—until finally he drops dead of exhaustion. But what if he had wagged his tail instead of baring his fangs?

The earthly home, in which we are surrounded by mirrors—what an extreme limitation of perception! Like an exaggerated parallel of the modern world, constricted by science. Like summoning up the Land of Ulro—the sad land of the imagination that has been disinherited by science, where objective necessity reigns and it is impossible "to credit marvels." The loss of the miraculous is connected with the progress of rationalism since the Enlightenment era. Of course, it is not about condemning the Enlightenment, or a return to the alleged idyll from before the scientific and technical revolution, nor about contrasting faith and reason. Such attempts, already made on more than one occasion, were a failure. Czesław

Miłosz believed that rescue might come not from accusing science, but from an entirely different image of the body and the world than the one offered us by eighteenth-century science and its offshoots to this day.

So in losing the "second space," in liberating ourselves from tradition, we would at the same time lose our sense of existing meaning—meaning that cannot simply be decreed according to our own will.

And what about the soul? What happened to it in the world that had lost its "second space" and become like the Land of Ulro? Here is how Adam Zagajewski answers this question in his poem entitled *The Soul*:

> *We know—or at least we have been told—*
> *that you do not exist at all, anywhere.*
> *And yet we still keep hearing your weary voice*
> *—in an echo, a complaint, in the letters we receive*
> *from Antigone in the Greek desert.*

The word "soul" is rarely heard nowadays among biologists or doctors. You would seek it in vain in the indexes of bulky volumes of psychiatry, or even psychology, not to mention internal medicine. Perhaps it appears in the occasional historical footnote. The word, as if mindful of its own nature . . . has evaporated. The "soul" has been replaced by the "self" and the "conscious self," or the "conscious mind." And at this moment the domain that from the start had always belonged to the philosophers began to shift towards the biologists and doctors. The majority believe that the conscious mind is located in the brain. Attempts have already been made to locate it within its defined structures. The mystery of the conscious mind has attracted some of the most brilliant intellects. It presents a challenge for those who have already reached the heights in other spheres of science, crowned with the Nobel Prize. And so Francis Crick, co-discoverer of the structure of DNA, or Gerard Edelman, who discovered the structure of immunoglobulin, have dropped the interests that took them so high to devote all their time to understanding the "self." But the "self" remains impenetrable and elusive, even though interesting new attempts to encapsulate it keep appearing. Some, like Christof Koch, seek consciousness in the material of the brain, in neurobiology, while others, like Douglas Hofstadter, deny its ontological reality and regard it as an illusion, "a mirage, a myth," generated by the complex machinery of the brain, accessible only at the highest level of thought, just as we can only comprehend the concept of pressure and temperature at a level of 10^{23} molecules, but not at the level of a single molecule. One of the more isolated views is held by British mathematician Roger Penrose, who says that these attempts are premature, because understanding the functions of the brain must be preceded by a revolution in physics, in comprehending the deepest structures of the world. Not even the greatest optimists imagine it would be possible to see the "self" with the use of stunning modern brain imaging techniques, even though they show how individual clusters of gray cells light up like colored islands in the dark ocean of the brain when they start to solve a task, when they listen, or count—in short, whenever they think.

However, is it right to narrow spiritual phenomena down to the conscious mind? After all, following the example of ultraviolet rays, "which are a light that possesses no brightness at all," very many spiritual phenomena "lack the glow of the conscious mind." The discovery of the unconscious mind is often ascribed to Freud, and yet long before him philosophers such as Aristotle or Schopenhauer referred to our unconscious desires, Goethe and Schiller sought the sources of literary creativity in the unconscious mind, and from the mid-nineteenth century onwards doctors, including some Polish ones, have devoted close attention and numerous treatises to it. Freud, however, made it the central idea in his teaching, and his originality relied on creating the concept of the displaced unconscious mind. The unconscious mind consists of urges and desires of which the ego rids itself by pushing them into oblivion because they conflict with reality and cause pangs of conscience. Once displaced, they are inaccessible to the cognition. The unconscious mind is "radically indifferent to reality," said Freud; logic is alien to it, as are the principles of non-contradiction and temporal sequence. Displacement concerns above all experiences with a sexual tinge from the period of early childhood. We are accustomed to calling the conscious, rational part of the psyche the "ego," our "self." It represents a relatively thin surface layer above the depths of the unconscious mind, which Freud called the "id." There is tension between them, a conflict, the "id" puts pressure on the "ego" — as if from below — with its blind urges. The conflict is revealed in our dreams, slips of the tongue and muddled memories. "One's own self is extremely well hidden from one's own self," said Nietzsche. According to this dictum we remain unrecognizable to ourselves, and our life is ruled by uncontrollable forces, hidden desires and passions. Yet we know a few things about ourselves that we cannot tell anyone. We realize that the person we keep quiet about is genuine — we are he or she. And the portrait that the world reflects back at us is just as much us as our inner image of ourselves, the one we never breathe a word about all our lives.

The concept of the conscious mind also creates "deep epistemological problems" and an evolutionary paradox. For if we accept, as the substantial majority of scientists do, that the experiences of the conscious mind originate in their entirety from present and past events, provided by way of the neurons, then every component of the conscious mind—and thus every shape, color, sound, thought, memory, intention, etc.—arises exclusively on this path. And so, if no magical transformation of all this information occurs in the brain, the conscious mind does not bring anything new to what the brain already contains. From this paradox the eminent Oxford neurophysiologist and former head of the Medical Research Council, Professor Colin Blakemore, concludes that "consciousness itself cannot have evolved by Darwinian selection. . . . Being conscious is an epiphenomenon."

One of the most famous American neurologists, Antonio Damasio, reckons there is a special center within our brains. It is not made up of cells that receive impressions from the surrounding world, transmitted by the senses. Instead it is formed by cells that receive signals coming from inside our bodies, including its furthest, deepest regions. These signals are transmitted along the nervous system or through the blood, like hormones. They are the basis for a special, moving map of the body that arises in the main center. The center in question is our "self," trapped as it were in the brain; it is the observer of events being played out on the stages of our inside, and the recipient of the feelings that accompany them. It passes them through the filters of the memory with which it is endowed. But isn't this image familiar to us from somewhere already? Isn't the "self," the spectator with an extensive memory shut inside us, by chance a little girl? The same Kore whom, as the Greeks believed, can be seen through the pupil of the eye? She listens to what we have to tell her, she reads the letters Antigone writes to us, and she smiles when she sees how our thought has come full circle in search of the soul, in order to reach her at last.

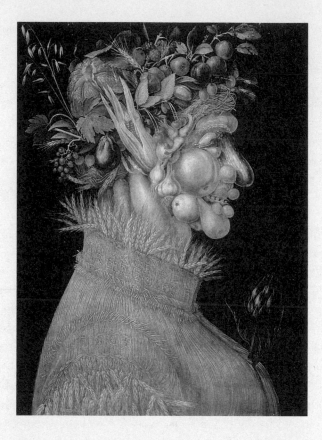

Giuseppe Arcimboldo
Summer, 1563
Kunsthistorisches Museum, Vienna

THE REFLECTED WORLD INSIDE US

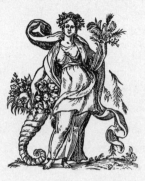

One time a mathematics student from Warsaw turned up at our hospital and told us the following story: it was summer, and he was traveling on a local train across a meadow, in which, far away by the woods, a horse was grazing. As the train rolled slowly past the field, our student felt his nose itching and began to sneeze, tears came to his eyes and before he had left the meadow behind him he was overcome with breathlessness. I had already seen it several times before: people who have come into a room where the day before, only briefly and for the first time ever, a cat has been playing, and have had a violent attack of asthma; others who have felt weak or even fallen to the floor as they accidentally breathed in penicillin prepared for injections; and I have even read about people who have been covered in hives at the mere sight of a flower in a picture. All of them had allergies. But can they really be as severe as in the story about the horse?

We performed the typical test in such cases, injecting an extract of horsehair under the skin. Just in case, we used a dilution ten thousand times weaker than recommended. After a few minutes the student's arm began to swell violently, and before we had time to realize, the swelling was up to his armpit. We hurriedly applied tourniquets to protect the student from the consequences of the reaction.

After a while we invited the patient to come in for desensitization treatment. For many weeks we gave him intracutaneous injections of increasingly concentrated extracts of horsehair. I do not have to say what sort of dilutions we started with, and what precautionary measures we took. We repeated this treatment the following years. The result was a remarkable lessening of his symptoms when exposed to horses, though our student never became a jockey.

In taking this action we were following in the footsteps of Mithridates VI, king of Pontus. This tyrant, famous for his cruelty, imprisoned his mother, killed his brother and married his sister. On his orders, issued from Ephesus, all the Italic tribes in Asia Minor were murdered in a single day, almost a hundred thousand people altogether. Mithridates was also a polyglot, who apparently knew twenty-two languages; he had a reputation as a patron of the arts and science and a friend of artists. Like all tyrants, he was afraid of being poisoned. Wishing to prevent this from happening, he conducted numerous experiments on his relatives and subjects to research poisons and their antidotes. Then every day for years, in ever-increasing doses, he drank an infusion containing the fifty-four most deadly poisons. His whole life he fought against Rome. Defeated by Antony in 66 BC, he never gave up the fight. But when his beloved son rose against him, he sank into despair and took a powerful draught of poison. However, it did not work — over the years the king's organism had become immune. Then he ordered a slave to run him through with a sword, and fell dead on the spot.

+++

Following Mithridates's example, we desensitize patients who are oversensitive to grass pollen, domestic dust, insects and animals. They are allergy sufferers. They are characterized by amazingly strong, dangerous reactions to substances in the outside world that are harmless to the rest of us. Desensitization was introduced into medicine in the early twentieth century. The first person to apply it on the North American continent was Robert A. Cooke. He had reasons for this—not just professional, but personal too. Cooke was brought up on a farm in New Jersey, and suffered from severe asthma from childhood onwards. Years later he recalled how he was "continuously ... inhaling little volcanoes of (burning) Himrod's asthma powder and vomiting from syrup of ipecac." Adrenalin was not yet known, nor was the word "allergy." When he went to school and lived in a boarding house, the asthma died down, but it returned whenever he went back to the farm, to his family home. He became convinced that it was triggered by contact with the horses kept in the stables. However, in those days it was hard to avoid horses. Towards the end of his studies, on a graduate traineeship, he was obliged to spend six months working as a traveling doctor for the emergency service. In the early twentieth century the New York ambulances were horse-drawn vehicles. Every trip to see a patient ended for Cooke in an attack of breathlessness. Before saving the patient he had to save himself, which he did with recently introduced shots of adrenalin. "I put as much adrenalin under my skin as any human being," wrote Cooke. But fate had an even bigger test in store for him. In 1907 he was helping to perform a tracheotomy. The operation was being carried out as a matter of urgency to save the life of a patient suffering from diphtheria, in those days a common and deadly illness. Just before the operation, as a prophylactic measure the operators were given an equine antitoxin against diphtheria, obtained by inoculating horses with diphtheria germs. Cooke fell to the ground on the spot and remained unconscious for ten hours. Is it any surprise that after these experiences Robert Cooke became fully preoccupied by the new discipline that was being born right before his eyes—allergology? He established the first big department for asthma sufferers in New York, made important clinical observations and ranked among the fathers of American allergology. "First be a doctor, then an allergist"—his favorite saying could apply to all medical specialties.

In treating allergies, and many other illnesses that have inflammation at their core (and, nowadays, even arteriosclerosis is regarded as an inflammation!), the most powerful defenses are hormones produced by the outer casing (the cortex) of some small endocrine glands, the adrenal glands. We call them corticosteroids. At the root of their discovery lay a question that in 1936 Philip Showalter Hench, an internist from the Mayo Clinic, put to chemist Edward Calvin Kendall. The question related to Hench's observation that in certain circumstances, a severe rheumatoid arthritis cures itself on its own without any drugs. Apparently Hench asked Kendall "if he could find a metabolite that was increased during pregnancies and during jaundice in view of his observation of the alteration of rheumatoid arthritis or asthma associated with these conditions." Kendall took up the challenge, and the rest is history. After more than ten years of research, he isolated this substance and demonstrated that it consists of hormones produced by the adrenal cortex. When the purified hormones were injected into some patients, one of the greatest miracles known to medicine occurred. People with twisted joints, groaning with pain and chained to their beds, stood up smiling, and people suffering from asthma, suffocating day and night, could breathe freely for the first time in their lives. In Stockholm there was little delay—two years later, both the questioner and the man he questioned received the Nobel Prize.

◆◆◆

There are no roses without thorns. Corticosteroids, which revolutionized medicine in the blink of an eye, carried some dangerous side effects. Some patients suddenly grew fat, others bled from the stomach, and yet others developed diabetes. Long years had to pass before we learned, and only partly, how to avoid these complications or neutralize them. So, not surprisingly, there has been no letup in the search for asthma drugs. The most original researcher was a young doctor named Roger Altounyan. He worked for a small British pharmaceuticals firm and tested new drugs on himself — not just once, or a few times, not just for a week or a month, but thousands of times over and for years on end. He had suffered from asthma during his medical studies and told himself he was a much more genuine model of the illness than the sensitized mice everyone tested potential pharmaceuticals on in those days.

He was allergic to many substances, including guinea pig hair, which became the main ingredient in his famous "hair soup." For four days he soaked the guinea pig hair, and then filtered the solution, thickened it and inhaled its vapors with the help of a nebulizer. Applied like this, the "hair soup" inevitably triggered asthma attacks in him, during which he made precise observations and took sensitive spirometric measurements. He conducted the experiments regularly, three times a week. He began in the early afternoon and finished in the evening. He attained a perfect repetition and standardization of his method, though sometimes the attacks he provoked were terribly dangerous and went on long into the night. Before administering his "soup" to himself, he would inhale new chemical compounds that were suspected of being able to weaken the attack or even prevent it. He was especially intrigued by extracts of an herb called *Ammi visnagae*, containing khellin, which was used to treat renal colic, because it expanded the smooth muscles of the ureters. Why did this particular plant, used in natural medicine for centuries by the peoples of the Mediterranean Sea basin, attract Altounyan so strongly? Did it remind him of the exemplary hospital in Aleppo, Syria, run by his doctor-father, where he even treated Lawrence of Arabia? In an eight-year period starting from 1957, Altounyan triggered over a thousand asthma attacks in himself and tested two hundred and two new chemical compounds. Finally, when he was sure he had hit upon the right form of khellin, he gave it to several patients and suffered a total failure—it had no effect at all. Only a few weeks later did he discover that for unknown reasons the incorrect chemical compound had been prepared for him. He repeated the experiment, this time with complete success. The drug, called Intal, was introduced to the market in the late 1960s and was a best seller for a long time in asthma treatment. Altounyan also designed an ingenious manual inhaler for controlling intake of the drug. Without a doubt, his experience as a pilot helped him with this—he flew fighter planes and bombers in the RAF, won the Air Force Cross and was a pilot instructor to the end of the war. The soul of the inhalator was a tiny propeller, and the device itself was called not a Spitfire, but . . . a Spinhaler.

I once spent a pleasant summer evening talking to Altounyan and his wife at my flat in Krakow. There opposite me sat someone extremely familiar to me from my childhood games, because a boy named Roger had been the hero of my favorite children's novel, *Swallows and Amazons*. With bated breath I used to follow in the wake of his little sailing boat as he and his peers set off on mysterious escapades to search for adventure and discover new lands. The amusements I had joined in with as a reader took place on Coniston Water in the Lake District in northern England, where Roger Altounyan's grandparents lived. Their friend and neighbor Arthur Ransome used to keep a close eye on the children's games on the water, and later depicted them in *Swallows and Amazons*.

Roger laughed at my account of those "joint" expeditions of ours from the distant past, but finally we had to go back to asthma.

I decided to take the bull by the horns, and asked him exactly how the drug he discovered works. "Why does it work in asthma?" And then he replied: "I'll give you an answer if you can tell me what asthma is."

Roger Altounyan found out what asthma is when, as a medical student at Cambridge, he went to see a doctor with the first attack of breathlessness he had ever had in his life. The doctor made his diagnosis and prescribed Phenobarbital, a soporific sedative, and ephedrine, which relaxes the smooth muscles. Then he pointed to his head and said: "The whole illness is in here." That was the prevailing belief at the time—the paradigm, as we would say nowadays. Doctors believed asthma was a disease of the central nervous system. Years later when Altounyan and I had our conversation at my flat, he was teaching his students in London and I was teaching mine in Krakow that at the heart of asthma lay a spasm of the muscles of the bronchial tubes, their oversensitive reaction to an extremely varied range of stimuli. No one said a word about the central nervous system. Nowadays, more than thirty years since that meeting, we teach something completely different: that asthma is a chronic inflammatory process of the airways. So here we have three diametrically different views of one of the most common illnesses. Doesn't medicine walk on shifting sands? A pragmatist would respond by saying that even if we have failed to capture the essence of the disease in a net of concepts, over the years we have taken great strides in treating asthma. It is true. Anyone trying to justify the conceptual difficulties and trouble in understanding asthma, and the variability of theories preached from the lectern, would certainly point out the diversity of the illness, which has been compared to love, because it is hard to define although everyone recognizes its symptoms.

For asthma is a thoroughly heterogeneous illness that finds its reflection in a wide variety of types, each individually identified within medicine. And so we speak of asthma that is allergic or non-allergic, seasonal or all-year-round, exercise-induced, brittle, nocturnal, professional or corticosteroid-resistant, as well as other kinds of asthma. These names alone indicate that we lack a single criterion of identity. The illness is variable and capricious — in some people it can run for a long time without any symptoms and not show up at all in the most sensitive clinical tests, while suffocating others for months, making it impossible for the doctor to seek the causes. In addition, the forms of asthma briefly mentioned here quite often change their shape, like clouds in the sky, combining common elements, and then turning into other ones again. One of the most common elements determining asthma is atopia. Watch out, Reader, because it could affect you too. Every fifth European or American has features of atopia. Fortunately, that is never synonymous with having the illness, but it indicates a very common occurrence of this genetic trait.

The word "atopia" was used in New York in the early 1920s to define a family tendency towards allergic reactions — unexpected and incomprehensible, and sometimes having a dramatic course, to the horror of the patient and those around him. These reactions and the related illnesses were completely baffling, even for medics who over the centuries have grown accustomed to the oddities of nature.

Atopos: the word is aptly chosen. It means different, separate, deviating from the norm, unusual. Alcibiades uses this word in Plato's *Symposium* to define Socrates. Were the New Yorkers who decided to introduce the word into medicine aware of its ancient history? We do not know, but we do know that at almost exactly the same time, two doctors in what was then the German city of Breslau conducted an experiment that half a century later gave rise to the isolation of the causative factor of atopia. Heinz Küstner,

who was starting work at the university's Hygiene Unit, told his
supervisor Otto Prausnitz that about fifteen minutes after eating cooked fish, he became covered in hives. As the same symptoms occurred in several of his blood relatives, the two scientists
began to suspect that the mystery might lie in the blood. So they
decided to give a subcutaneous injection of several drops of Küstner's blood serum to Prausnitz, who ate fish with relish and no difficulty. Nothing happened. But when twenty-four hours later they
injected a trace of extract of cooked fish in the same spot, his arm
went red and became covered in hives. Other healthy volunteers
reacted in a similar way. Thus the sensitivity could be transferred to
a healthy person, though not to guinea pigs. The two experimenters drew the conclusion that a person who is sensitive to fish carries
antibodies in the blood (which they named precipitins) against fish
antigens. Precipitins injected into a healthy person attach themselves under the skin (nowadays, we know that they fix onto the
membrane of special "explosive" cells called mastocytes), and wait
for the antigen that is an extract of fish meat to come through.
Then they combine with these antigens to cause an explosive reaction. Precipitins proved extremely difficult to isolate; it took forty-
five years for them to be obtained, highly purified, from the blood.
They were found to be a protein in the immunoglobulin group,
and were identified with the letter E. Thus atopia is a genetic tendency towards overproduction of immunoglobulin E. Precipitins
are often aimed at common antigens, and when additional factors
are at work, they can lead to the development of hay fever, hives or
asthma. Our math student and Doctor Cooke, who were both so
severely allergic to horses, must have been producing special antibodies against equine tissues in high concentrations, whereas hay
fever sufferers or those who are allergic to dust produce immunoglobulin E against the pollen from grasses, weeds and some trees.

◆◆◆

It is possible to cure illnesses using antibodies. Emil von Behring adopted this idea: by injecting animals with diphtheria bacteria, he then obtained special antibodies from them that inactivated these bacteria. Given to patients, they saved their lives at a severe stage of the illness, which often ended in death otherwise. For this research, in 1901 Behring was the first person in history to win the Nobel Prize for medicine. In its statement, the Nobel Committee wrote that he had "placed in the hands of the physician a victorious weapon against illness and deaths." The eminent continuer of this research, Paul Ehrlich, said that "the immune substances . . . in the manner of magic bullets, seek out the enemy." Moved by these events, George Bernard Shaw wrote a play called *The Doctor's Dilemma*, in which the title hero claims that the future of scientific therapy belongs to immunology, whereas "drugs are a delusion."

The antibodies acquired by inoculating horses and other animals were heterogeneous, however, and as a result they sometimes caused highly allergic reactions in the patients. Scholars and doctors began to dream of producing pure immunoglobulins on a large scale. To make this dream come true, it proved helpful to introduce the in vitro cultivation of cells of a particular tumor (multiple myeloma, or plasmacytoma), which produces immunoglobulins, but ones that are devoid of immunological properties. In the mid-1960s an ingenious technique was devised for combining two cells into one. And so from one myeloma cell and one immune system cell that secretes a specific immunoglobulin, a hybrid was obtained that produced an unlimited quantity of pure, homogeneous antibodies of a defined specificity. They were called monoclonal antibodies. Efforts began to seek applications for them in diagnostics and therapy. As always, the first success boosted the research. Rituximab, a drug used to treat non-Hodgkin's lymphoma—malignant tumors in the lymphatic system—proved a spectacular success. Several others followed. More and more often, instead of the full antibodies, which are long particles shaped like the letter Y, small pieces of them are applied. So, for example, a short section of antibody is fastened onto an anti-cancer drug, which recognizes the "signatures" of tumors, in other words, the individual receptors on their surface. Thus the antibodies become a navigator, the warhead for a shell full of the drug, which they guide accurately to its target. There are hundreds of these and similar antibodies in pre-clinical or clinical trials. Although they have not yet become a magic weapon, if he were still alive George Bernard Shaw could boldly write his next play about them.

Over the last few pages the words "antigen" and "antibody" have appeared a number of times. Alongside lymphocytes, they are the actors on the stage of this chapter, which talks about allergy as derived from the study of immunity, in other words, immunology. The antigen comes to us from the outside world and encounters an antibody produced by the lymphocytes, which extinguishes and inactivates it. We call the sub-group of antigens that trigger allergy "allergens." They are a small part of a vast set, including bacteria, viruses and everything else that is alien to us, or not part of our "self." And the "self" is whatever the immune system recognizes as its own, as belonging to its body. This distinction protects us from being invaded by the world, and is crucial to our existence. Yet there are situations in which the doctor uses powerful drugs to stupefy the immune system. So it is in transplant medicine, where we put glasses on the immune system to make it start to see an alien, transplanted organ as its own. Then instead of sending millions of killer cells to attack the new arrival, it accepts it as an integral part of its body. The range of organs or tissues being transplanted is growing rapidly, as well as the number of operations. The most spectacular transplants involve the heart. How can we fail to admire forty-two-year-old American Kelly Parking, who eight years after receiving a new heart climbed to the top of the Matterhorn and came down again, without any medical care? Or the Canadian man who had a heart transplant at the age of twenty-six, and twenty years later completed the Olympic triathlon distance in three hours and twenty minutes, coming seventy-fifth out of a hundred and twenty-six starters?

Of course, a transplant carries risks. In 1968 Andrzej Wajda made an extremely funny comedic film about them, with the English title *Roly Poly*. It was based on a story by Stanisław Lem, and the main role was played by Bogumił Kobiela. The hero is a race car driver who, after lots of accidents in car races, has various organ transplants. We see his psyche gradually changing, until in the final scene, when the word "bone" crops up in the conversation, he attacks the man who said it and bites his hand, because he has some organs taken from a dog inside him too. In a foreword added to this novella much more recently, Lem explained that over twenty-five years ago he could not have known that a transplant from dog to man is impossible. But he seemed not to have noticed (though can he really have failed to notice anything?) that he foresaw how features transfer from donor to recipient with amazing insight. Not long ago, a leukemia patient was described as having acquired hay fever along with a bone marrow transplant; he had never suffered from it before, but it was the bane of the donor's life. However, considering the bone marrow saved his life, perhaps he found it easy to come to terms with the hay fever, which turned up every spring from then on.

The definition of the "self"—which in psychology has replaced the soul, without removing the semantic, physiological and existential problems related to it—in terms of immunology is simple.

Let us repeat: the "self" is whatever the immune system accepts as its own, as belonging to its body. All right, but what about the rest of the world? How do we recognize it? How do we keep it at a distance? How do we guarantee this unimaginable wealth of anti-bodies, each of which is directed only and exclusively at one single antigen among billions?

For decades it was believed that the antibodies we carry inside us — whether free ones in the form of gamma-globulin, or those anchored in the lymphocytes — form their individuality in an encounter with an alien antigen when it gets inside us. In other words, we thought they were characterized by flexibility, or plasticity, as if they were made of plasticine, on which an alien invader (the antigen) then stamped its mark and molded them to make them fit it exactly, as a key fits a lock. And then, by multiplying, they bonded with it closely and inactivated it.

This theory reached its apogee in the 1950s. It was the paradigm supported by the great Linus Pauling, among others, who had already won two Nobel Prizes by then, but it collapsed like a house of cards thanks to a Dane named Niels Jerne. He worked for a Copenhagen producer of serums and inoculations, where he was involved with anti-diphtheria serums. When a horse was inoculated with diphtheria germs, its large organism produced significant amounts of antibodies, which were then given to patients as a serum — such as Cooke was given, we remember, who was sensitive to horses and almost died. Jerne's task was to standardize immunological serums. He hit upon a fundamental problem for standardization: a lack of proportion between successive dilutions of serums and the strength of their action. Each time the dilutions came out slightly different. Then he formed a hypothesis that the equine serums he was testing contained special antibodies before the horse was inoculated. The inoculation merely caused a tremendous multiplication of these antibodies. Then Jerne demonstrated that his supposition was true. The phenomenon he discovered could have two explanations. The first one was obvious and convincing: earlier on, the horse had already come across the bacteria with which it was later inoculated, and preserved the memory of that contact in the form of a small number of antibodies in its blood. This seemed all the more obvious since horses and other animals used in experiments were especially prone to exposure to bacteria. Don't we all carry such memories inside from unnoticed encounters with bacteria or viruses?

But Jerne thought of another eventuality. Perhaps, he wrote, the horse's or man's animal system comes into the world equipped with antibodies against *all* possible microorganisms? Maybe it has them ready in advance, before encountering any potential invader? And this proved to be the truth; eventually it was sealed with a Nobel Prize. And so the immune system is able to react individually to practically every microorganism, and moreover, to every antigen in the world around us, because it is suitably equipped for this purpose in the mother's womb. Hundreds of millions of B lymphocytes, each with a different antibody on the surface, are just waiting to encounter their antigens. The individuality of these antibodies does not have to be great, just enough to bond to the antigen in the first place. It rapidly increases within the progeny of those first lymphocytes. In recent years scientists have explained the molecular mechanism of this seemingly paradoxical phenomenon; we have a limited yet fairly large number of genes at our disposal, and with them we are able to produce billions of different antibodies.

How is such a highly original theory born? Where does the inspiration come from? Ten years after making this discovery, Jerne described an evening in Copenhagen, when he was on his way home from the laboratory. He was considering how 10^{17} gammaglobulin particles are able to provide a specificity of antibodies. Before reaching home the theory now familiar to us had fallen into place. Can it have been the influence of Søren Kierkegaard, his favorite Danish philosopher, whom he often read? Jerne posed this question but did not give a definitive answer. He merely offered the comment that if, in a text by Kierkegaard, instead of the word "truth" we were to put the words "antibodies' ability to synthesize," then the text changes into an expression of his theory. Here is the text: "Can the truth [the capability to synthesize an antibody] be learned? If so, it must be assumed not to pre-exist; to be learned, it must be acquired. We are thus confronted with the difficulty to which Socrates calls attention in *Meno*, ... namely, that it makes as little sense to search for what one does not know as to search for what one knows; what one knows, one cannot search for, since one knows it already, and what one does not know, one cannot search for, since one does not even know what to search for. Socrates resolves this difficulty by postulating that learning is nothing but recollection. The truth [the capability to synthesize an antibody] cannot be brought in, but was already inherent."

How Platonic Jerne's theory sounds in this context! Therefore only a fraction of knowledge reaches us from the outside world. The organism does not experience anything new when it comes into contact with an antigen. It is all inside us already. In the language of molecular biology, it is impossible to impose information about the synthesis of antibodies on DNA; this knowledge is already contained within it.

Attempts have also been made to find the qualities in Jerne's personality that influenced his adoption of this unexpected, fantastical, but true concept. This drew attention to the fact that long before making his discovery, he had noticed that as a human being he had a large number of ready psychological reactions stored up at his disposal, which he used in order to face the world. Nietzsche would surely have applauded this reasoning, because he wrote: "Gradually it has become clear to me what every great philosophy so far has been: namely, the personal confession of its author and a kind of involuntary and unconscious memoir."

When we think of Jerne's theory — its scientific name is clonal selection — we are overcome with admiration and amazement, similar to what we feel as we gaze at a starry sky. This theory implies a connection with the starry sky and also with the closer world around us. It tells us that we are its reflection. The wise men and great poets sensed this, and their intuition anticipated science. Origen, the most famous theologian of the East, who "built the edifice of Christian knowledge with Greek bonding," said: "Understand that you are another world in miniature and that in you are the sun, the moon, and also the stars." Leibniz reckoned that any "individual substance" must contain a complete image of the universe, like a seed that conceals inside (if only as an image) the entire being that will later grow from it. Whereas Rainer Maria Rilke believed we are so similar to this world that if we were to sit still and keep quiet, it would be impossible to tell us apart from it. And so we have nothing to fear. It is not inconceivable, he says, that it is just as with those dragons from the oldest myths known to man, which at a decisive moment change into princesses. "Perhaps all the dragons of our life are princesses, who are only waiting to see us once beautiful and brave." And finally Czesław Miłosz, who wrote: "Perhaps the world was created by the Good Lord to reflect itself in the infinite number of eyes of living creatures, or, what is more probable, in the infinite number of human consciousnesses."

I imagine that the molecules that form antibodies, in bonding with an antigen, must vibrate according to the laws of physics, and thus they resound inside us. So, as in music, all together they create a canon, a mirror image canon, in which the second, following voice imitates the first voice perfectly. So perhaps we are playing the canon of the universe? And perhaps, like the harmony of the celestial spheres, this music resounds inside each of us, but none of us can hear it, except for the poets, to whom certain themes and inner rhythms break through from the depths of the body and dictate the meter of the poetry to them like a musical daemon. From the moment we are born we carry the world inside us. We are its matrix, and if the world were ever to perish, it could find itself within us and regenerate from us.

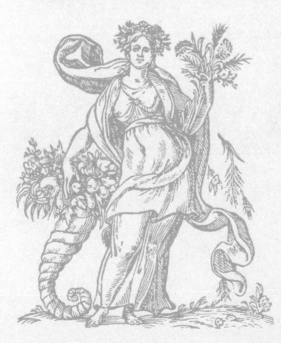

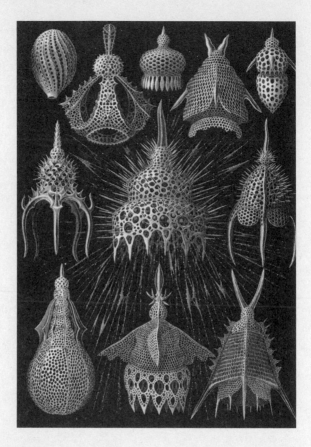

Ernst Haeckel
Cystoidea
An illustration from the book *Kunstformen der Natur,* 1904

THE ARCANA OF ART AND THE
RIGORS OF SCIENCE

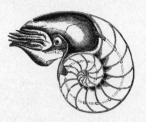

In Mikhail Bulgakov's novel *The Master and Margarita* there is a scene where Christ, who in this story is called Yehuda Ha-Notsri, is standing before Pontius Pilate. All morning the Procurator of Judea has been suffering from a painful headache. He has a hemicrania, a migraine, which he has never confessed to anyone. Then comes the famous question: "What is truth?"

Ha-Notsri replies: "At this moment the truth is chiefly that your head is aching and aching so hard that you are having cowardly thoughts about death.... But the pain will stop soon and your headache will go."

"Tell me," says Pilate softly in Latin, "are you a great physician?"

Here we have an instant diagnosis, read from the patient's face—an attribute of divinity, of course. But also the ideal to which the doctor should aspire. Does this connotation sound arrogant or even blasphemous? I do not think so. In various world religions the gods have the power to pervade man, to look into his deepest secrets, as part of the gift of healing and reviving, skills in the sphere of the miraculous. The Bible gives us some examples. And did not

Asclepius have the art of resurrecting the dead? Who other than Isis, the most powerful goddess of ancient Egypt, brought Osiris back to life, although he had been chopped to bits? Echoes of these miraculous diagnoses and cures lie hidden in the doctor's vocation.

The desire to perform a miracle, to break the chains of everyday normality, to be free of the laws that bind us, was there at the dawn of medicine. This was what magic was for — the common stem from which both medicine and art originate. Magic was a system based on the omnipotence of the word: "A correctly uttered magic spell can bring health or death, rain or drought, call up the spirits or reveal the future." At a later point in time the art of the word, aided by experience, was joined by a second element: thought, an attempt to understand. From then on reason became a companion to the art of healing, and went along with it for thousands of years, until it produced science, which led to the flourish of biology and medicine. Naturally, it influenced the art of healing, though it has never supplanted or replaced it. Nowadays, of course, in the era of technological revolution, we sometimes tend to assume it has.

Efforts to understand the nature of things came earlier. It was at the turn of the seventh and sixth centuries BC that practical skills were converted into scientific theory. This was apparently achieved, in the Greek colonies on the coast of Asia Minor, by one of seven wise men, Thales of Miletus. Whenever the Greek philosophers sought their progenitor, they looked back in time and came to him. This was as far as they could go into the past — Thales was the first person to think of the unity of the universe, because the object of his investigations was nature. He was chiefly interested in its origins, so he asked from what bodies (nowadays, we would say matter) it had hatched and developed. Finding an answer was hopelessly difficult, because how could Thales know what was there at the beginning of the world? However, he deserves credit not for providing answers, but for posing questions, something we value highly in science to this day. He also aspired to explaining some phenomena. This had already been done by mythology before him, but the point is that his method of explaining was different.

A story has survived about him that tells how one night he was in the garden, staring at the stars; absorbed by his observations; he was so deeply lost in thought that he fell into a well. Then he heard laughter — loud, resonant laughter. It was a Thracian servant girl, who was laughing at him for seeking paths in the sky, but failing to walk the Earth.

A few years later, in nearby Ephesus, a memorable scene took place. It was night, and there in the temple before the goddess stood Heraclitus. He had brought the fruits of his life's work, a great book of wisdom. The goddess looked at the visitor. A copy of her statue, kept at the Naples Museum, allows us to envisage this scene more vividly. Entirely made of black wood, she has collars and necklaces around her neck and is wrapped in ethereal robes; from the waist down she is encased in cloth, richly adorned with pictures of flora and fauna. She is stuck inside it, as in a box, with only the tips of her black toes protruding. Her hands are turned outwards towards the visitor, as if she wants to greet him, present or show something to him. Her torso is naked, covered in several rows of ample breasts. She is Artemis, equated with the Egyptian Isis, the goddess of nature, a powerful queen of the Mediterranean world and the source of creative force — the Mother of all Nature, as Apuleius calls her. She looms out of the darkness of prehistory — mysterious, strange and inscrutable. We see her, centuries later, in pictures, frescoes and statues. In Raphael's work she has been doubled and supports both sides of the throne of Philosophy in the fresco called

The School of Athens on the vault of the Stanza della Segnatura in the Vatican Palace. She adorns the covers of famous books by Antony van Leeuwenhoek, whose treatise on microscopy describes the *interiora rerum*, the insides of things. She opens an eighteenth-century French translation of Lucretius's *De Rerum Natura*, published at the Sorbonne as *De la Nature des Choses*. As drawn by Bertel Thorvaldsen, she occupies the title page of a work that Alexander von Humboldt gave to Goethe. And finally she gazes as us from the cover of a long epic poem by Erasmus Darwin, grandfather of Charles, *The Temple of Nature, or, the Origin of Society*. On these and many other images the veil covering her has been drawn aside or even removed. This is done by the hand of Apollo, the spirit of Epictetus or, more and more often as the centuries go by, Science, represented as her high priestess. And so the secrets of Nature are discovered. There before us stands the naked truth.

We do not know if Artemis-Isis drew aside the hem of her veil before Heraclitus in the temple. Nor do we know the title of the work he laid at her feet. However, we do have reason to believe it contained the powerful concepts that he introduced into philosophy: the idea of divine reason pervading an ever-changing world full of contrasts. There in the temple he spoke the words written in his book, saying: "Nature likes to hide" (φύσις κρύπτεσθαι φιλεῖ). This laconic remark, pregnant with meaning, was the object of numerous interpretations. What did "Nature" mean to Heraclitus? It does not seem to have signified a large set of natural phenomena subject to laws. This meaning took shape later on. Whereas he may have thought of nature as meaning the essence of things, their main constitutional feature. And he may also have thought about the origin of things, about their beginnings, and how they came to be. Experts on ancient Greek maintain that for Heraclitus "the word

Φύσις (*phusis*) could designate birth, while the word κρύπτεσθαι (*kruptesthai*), for its part, could evoke disappearance or death." And so this aphorism may have concealed Heraclitus's characteristic amazement at the transience of things and people, who come into being and disappear, are born, and then die. This is the firm belief that the structure of the world is woven from contradictory though mutually supporting elements. The Stoics related his words to the gods, hidden within myths. Later on they served as explanations for the difficulties of the natural sciences, justified the exegesis of biblical texts or defended pagan beliefs and pointed out the violence inflicted on Nature by the mechanization of the world. The closer to the modern day, the more the mysteries hidden behind Isis's veil came to be related to the mystery of existence.

Heraclitus's words, like Nature of whom they spoke, were hidden within themselves. They were an enigmatic aphorism, a riddle, a wise saying from ancient Greece, sounding like a prophecy by the Delphic oracle. They formed an extremely powerful metaphor that was preserved in language. They shaped the concept of Nature, of which we are actually a part; they spoke of discovering her laws and seeking the truth about the character of science. And there were scholars, including Immanuel Kant and especially Francis Bacon, who put Nature before a tribunal, announcing that the truth should be wrung out of her, "under the torture of experiments." At the other extreme stood Goethe, who warned of the danger concealed behind the veil of "Nature the Sphinx." Whereas Nietzsche, jokingly pointing out that decency demands us not to want to see everything naked, wrote: "One should have more respect for the *bashfulness* with which nature has hidden behind riddles and iridescent uncertainties." And then he added: "Perhaps truth is a woman who has grounds for not showing her grounds?"

In the *Hippocratic Corpus*, dating from the fifth century BC, we read that to know Nature, "one cannot know anything certain . . .

from any other quarter than from medicine," and that "this knowledge is to be attained when one comprehends the whole subject of medicine properly, but not until then; and I say that this history shows what man is, by what causes he was made, and other things accurately." The author was convinced that by means of art one could wring signs out of Nature, clinical symptoms — but "without damage." In these words we hear Greek moderation and the Hippocratic command, "Above all do no harm" (*Primum non nocere*). "Because moderation," as Pythagoras said, "means not doing harm."

In the Musée Royal des Beaux Arts in Brussels there is a painting by Pieter Brueghel the Elder called *The Fall of Icarus*. It is painted in shades of green, reflecting the illuminated green of the sea picking up flashes of the sun, which is setting beyond the horizon. We gaze at the sea from the gentle shore above a small bay. In the foreground a ploughman is following his plough, lower down a shepherd is tending his sheep and a fisherman is leaning forwards right at the water's edge. An elaborate three-masted ship is sailing across the bay. The fall of Icarus is not disturbing this peaceful scene. Close to the shore, between the ship and the fisherman, all we can see of the boy who has fallen into the sea is his legs sticking out of the surface and an outstretched hand. There are a few feathers floating in the air. No one seems surprised; no one is taking any notice or reacting. Except perhaps a partridge that has perched on a branch over the water behind the fisherman's back, and has fixed its gaze on the disappearing boy. This indifference, this lack of understanding, astounds W.H. Auden:

> *In Brueghel's Icarus, for instance: how everything turns away*
> *Quite leisurely from the disaster; the ploughman may*
> *Have heard the splash, the forsaken cry,*

But for him it was not an important failure; the sun shone
As it had to on the white legs disappearing into the green
Water; and the expensive delicate ship that must have seen
Something amazing, a boy falling out of the sky,
had somewhere to get to and sailed calmly on.

Icarus does not die alone; he dies among people. Brueghel found a brilliant way to express the truth about man, about "the phenomenon of the world's indifference, which belongs to fundamental experiences." We do not want to see suffering, so we turn our backs on misfortune. It always comes at the wrong time; it obstructs and nags like a thorn, even though it is not stuck under our skin. It catches us off guard. And only the doctor, the nurse or the hospital chaplain comes out early to meet it. They have to preserve their sensitivity to avoid becoming participants in the scene depicted by Brueghel.

Sensitivity has a special place in medicine. On the one hand, as doctors, we have to put on a layer of armor; otherwise, we would never be able to cope with all the misery and suffering around us. Otherwise, the doctor would start to cry with the patients, after an hour's work he would be good for nothing and the surgeon would break down at the operating table. We put on this armor every day, both doctors and nurses.

On the other hand it carries a risk, because over time it can impose a lack of empathy, a feeling of indifference. But in fact it is emotion that sends the first impulse to stir the doctor into action. I imagine, Reader, that if we were walking along together, and someone were to fall over, we would both instantly bend down to give him a hand and raise him to his feet; at most, I might know a bit more about how to help him. That's an ordinary, human reflex, isn't it? Something is bound to react inside us. It should be automatic, but life does not depend on reflex responses alone, because we are not machines. You have to nurture this sensitivity in your-self — to have a sensitive heart. It is not often talked about, because sensitivities are mainly expected from artists. Perhaps the connec-tions between medicine and art are apparent at this level too.

Being sensitive enables us to be open towards another person, ready to admit him. The sick "open up spaces for mercy. By their illness and suffering they call forth acts of mercy and create the possibility for accomplishing them." But how difficult they can be! Imagine it is night-time, and the ambulance brings in yet another gibbering, drunken patient. Or the hospital corridor is teeming with people in wet coats who have been waiting hours to be admit-ted and examined. They are fed up to the back teeth, but are they the only ones? And yet how much each of them can bring into our lives! What a happy surprise there is in store for us when a quiet person, whom we have looked down on in our arrogant way, turns out to be wonderful! I once had an experience of this kind, and it had a medical connection.

It happened during the 1981–1983 martial law period in Poland, which was also known as "the Poland-Jaruzelski War." In Soli-darity we prepared a First of May counter-demonstration to spite WRON — the Military Council for National Salvation, as the rul-ing body headed by General Jaruzelski was called. The Polish word *wrona* also means "crow," so people kept singing street songs about "the green crow," because of the green military uniforms worn by its leaders, the people responsible for martial law, as well as their mouthpieces, the television presenters.

It was 1 May 1983, and so for May Day the authorities had orga-nized speeches in support of martial law in Krakow Marketplace, next to the Town Hall Tower. The Soviet consul and some other government people were already on the tribune. The clock struck ten, and from the forest of loudspeakers surrounding the Marketplace came a solemn announcement: General Jaruzelski, First Secretary of the Central Committee of the Polish United Workers' Party, president of the Council of Ministers and chairman of WRON, was going to make a speech. There was a moment of silence and anticipation, but instead of the general's voice from the loudspeakers out came ... a long, raucous noise of crows cawing. It had worked! The cawing filled the Marketplace, echoing down the neighboring streets and carrying a long way, as if it were only going to stop at the much-hated headquarters of WRON, in Warsaw. Hordes of people just then emerging from Saint Mary's church were overcome with a frenzy of joy. In a broad wave we set off towards the party tribune, which the dignitaries were starting to abandon in confusion. We had no bad intentions; we were just carried away by joy and elation. However, I did not know that the head of the procession was being filmed by hidden cameras. A few days later, in Warsaw, I was dismissed from my job as deputy vice-chancellor of the Medical Academy and forbidden to teach my classes. "And now," said the Minister of Health, "you can look forward to a trial for inciting riots against the people's authority." Crowds of Cracovians came to the trial. We stalled for time, because there was talk of an amnesty likely to coincide with the approaching anniversary of the PKWN Manifesto on 22 July (the PKWN was the Polish Committee of National Liberation, a Soviet-sponsored body that governed areas of Poland newly liberated from German occupation in 1944).

Finally, the decisive moment came: identification of the accused on the basis of some photographs, apparently not in very sharp focus. A witness was brought into the courtroom, and in came Captain Mieczysław Dec from the Medical Academy's Military

Studies department, whose head was the academy's military commissar — during martial law Jaruzelski imposed one on every academic institution, to keep an eye on their senior staff. "Oh no, it's him — it couldn't be worse," I thought. And back came the memory of the morning long ago when he had caught three of us medical students playing cards on the back bench during a talk in the jampacked Military Studies lecture hall. An hour later we were standing at the front of the assembly. "What have you got to say?" asked Lieutenant Dec. "The ace of hearts is missing, Sir," replied my friend Janek, holding our pack of cards that had just been returned to him.

Do I have to write what happened after that? Do I have to say that he could never forget us and our arrogance for all the years that followed? Because we had Military Studies classes once a week for the entire course of our medical studies.

And here he was in the courtroom, years later, in a captain's uniform by now, as a witness before the tribunal. One of the three judges showed him the photographs and asked: "Who do you recognize here?" After a long pause the Captain replied: "I can't see, I didn't bring my glasses — I didn't know they'd be needed." "Take mine!" cried the judge, removing his glasses from his nose. The Captain calmly took them, tried them and replied: "Too weak." They had to take a break in the trial. And although I was eventually convicted, it happened with some delay, three days before the amnesty, and I managed to avoid prison. None of us had expected such courage and ingenuity on the part of the captain, who took a very big risk. I have great admiration for him to this day.

This story had a third and final act. It was 1990, and I was starting a new job as vice-chancellor of the Medical Academy, having been freely elected to the post after the fall of communism. An application came in for a small salary raise before retirement, which the applicant was due to take soon. It was signed "Colonel Dec."

Dec? I had not seen him since that day at the trial. I had thought of meeting with him to say thank you, but I knew that at the time it would have been incriminating for him, and later on ... I forgot. "Please ask the Colonel to come and see me," I said to the office manager, who shot me a glance from over a pile of correspondence without hiding her surprise. The matter was self-evident, trivial, the raise was due...

There we sat face-to-face. "Colonel," I said, "after all these years I want to say thank you and tell you how much I admire your courage." For a while he said nothing, and then he looked me in the eye and quietly asked: "Citizen Vice-Chancellor, may I have permission to go now, Sir?" "Colonel," I boomed, "permission granted!" He stood straight as a ramrod and clicked his heels together. About turn, and Colonel — Captain — Lieutenant Dec left the final act of the story that had brought us together.

This tale in three parts reminds me of the Solidarity union we formed and that we lived by throughout the 1980s. We were the latest generation of Poles to fight for independence, a fact that none of us doubted in the slightest. Of course, the words "trade unions" were always tripping off our tongues, but it was clear the aim was liberation. We had gulped down the breath of freedom when Solidarity first erupted. And even in the later, increasingly dismal 1980s, when the regime did everything it could to "atomize" society, we experienced the "unity of hearts" we heard about from our Pope, without whom none of it would have happened. It was to him, to the Vatican, that I twice flew from Krakow in 1981. One time a friend came with me, a brilliant scholar, who was later to prove his integrity during martial law. But at that point, when there were shortages of everything in Poland, and western universities were opening their doors to us, he was troubled by the question of whether to stay in the West. He sought an answer from the Pope, and asked the question. John Paul II looked deep into his eyes and answered: "Isn't it already enough that I have had to stay here?"

In 1984, a renowned Italian professor of pharmacology named Rodolfo Paoletti sought me out, and in a concerned tone spent a long time explaining: "Give it a rest. You have no chance at all. You are in for the fate of the Balkans under the Turks — Soviet occupation for the next three centuries. Better send your children to Russian schools." Although his motives were well-meant and realistic, I replied with the traditional Italian bent elbow. Did any of us really expect communism to collapse in our lifetime? But it did, and we won. The independence that followed proved difficult, and our everyday world was crippled. The national capacity for resistance, the ability to put up opposition, ceased to be of any use. Suddenly we felt a lack of people — in politics, the courts and schools; in every area of life — following the terrible devastation of war, as well as the devastation that had gone on for decades ever since the war had ended. Personal interests began to grow, and unrestrained selfishness. We soon came to believe that "triumph over the powers of evil does not make a good person of anyone," as Joseph Brodsky put it. If only we had had as much success in the years of work on internal renewal as we did with independence.

For those of us living here in the 1980s, medicine was different. Sometimes a patient on a hospital ward would steal his neighbor's medicine because he knew there was not enough of it for him. The faucets were always disappearing, because they were unattainable in the city. Not to mention that food was apportioned on ration cards, or that toilet paper was always in short supply all over the country, and then there was the gray, ashen dust that got into everything — it was under our eyelids, between our teeth, in the hospital, on the streets and in the houses. We organized the distribution of medicines and clothes that humanitarian organizations sent by truck from abroad (it was French and German people in particular who brought them to Krakow, brave, courageous men and women who subjected themselves to various forms of mortification), we bandaged and hid people who had been injured in street demonstrations, we printed and distributed leaflets and forbidden books and we built up an underground organization at the local and national level. For many of us, there was nothing more important than Solidarity.

But, meanwhile, in the world outside medicine did not stop and wait for us. It was busy making amazing advances and tackling illnesses. It was probing deep inside the human body, turning more and more often towards the exact sciences in order to understand its own discoveries.

In the past two centuries the final judgment on illness was played out on the stage of the *theatrum anatomicum*. The autopsy, supported by microscope research, established a verdict that was irrevocable. It confirmed, or refuted, the clinical diagnosis, revealing new areas of knowledge of mankind. This was still the case in our grandfathers' and fathers' day. But by the time I was a student, biochemistry was taking the lead, and the causes of illnesses were being discerned in the transformation of chemical compounds during metabolism and in its disorders. Increasingly often, mysteries were being unearthed from inside the human body — without opening it up. Methods for producing images of the organs flourished. The large-scale collection of tissue samples from live patients also began, to be used to recreate the picture of an illness. Today, several decades on, we seek explanations for the phenomena occurring in the human body at the molecular level, by examining the particles that form proteins and DNA ... And so from inspecting the entire body we are penetrating deeper and deeper, into the ever tinier elements that form each of us. What may be in store for us at the deepest level? Mathematical equations that describe the physical world of man — that is how some would answer.

It is not the first time doctors have turned to mathematics. In the seventeenth century the connection between these two disciplines seemed so close that on the title pages of their works (and also on their epitaphs), many doctors wrote the honorable title *"medicus mathematicus"* after their names. So, for example, at Saint Wojciech's church in Krakow, on a late Renaissance tombstone we read: *"Valentino Fontano medico math[e-matico].""* Shakespeare calls the doctor who examines Lady Macbeth as she tries to wash the blood from her hands in a sleepwalking trance a "Doctor of Physics," and in my childhood the old people in Subcarpathia used to say "physicist" instead of "doctor."

Where did it come from? From a fascination with the progress of mathematics, physics and mechanics — from admiration for Newton, Descartes and William Harvey. The symbol of a turning point in science was Galileo. Until then, to explain the phenomena of nature, scholars simply cited the traditional authorities. From his time onwards they began to rely on their own observations and experiments. Admiration for Galileo became so widespread that in 1737, when his remains were transported to the upper nave of Santa Croce church in Florence, the middle finger of his right hand was separated from the rest of his body to be kept as a holy relic. Now it is displayed in the Museo di Storia della Scienza. On the cylindrical alabaster foot of the chalice in which it lies is the inscription: "Do not spurn the remains of this finger, whose right hand showed mortals paths on the horizon and celestial bodies never seen before." Indeed, "we see . . . Galileo's finger dabbling in all our current scientific pies." Galileo was also the spiritual father of the entire schools of iatromechanics and iatromathematics, which in the sixteenth and seventeenth centuries tried to make medicine into an exact science.

In this period a doctor and professor in Padua and Venice named Santorio Santorio constructed not only thermometers, pulsimeters and hygrometers, but also scales so large that "he sat in them himself, and even lived there (with a bed, a desk, etc.), while weighing and measuring everything, like Galileo." In time, these ideas and measurements of his led to the study of metabolism. Santorio's pupils — the iatrophysicists, worked on the mechanics of the body, comparing the blood circulation system to hydraulic machines and reckoning the nerves are small tubes in which juices circulate.

But does biology, and with it medicine, have its own universal laws? Or is that the exclusive domain of physics? The views of biologists and physicists have taken a different shape in this regard. Let us consider the laws of Mendel, the so-called central dogma of genetics, or the "law" of natural selection. Exceptions to these laws have not caused alarm or sent biologists back to the drawing board to formulate new laws that cover the exceptions. Instead, they have come to be a reminder of how complex biology really is.

Nowadays, however, when physicists, mathematicians, IT experts and engineers are sought out by biologists and doctors, when university systems biology departments are springing up like mushrooms after rain, questions about principles and laws are taking on practical significance. Can one really speak of the emerging principles, or maybe even laws, of networks? Of a kind that would cover some incredibly complex systems, such as metabolic reactions, or the paths of signals inside a cell? Can there really be a "universal architecture," representing "one of the very few universal mathematical laws of life"?

Perhaps, as they enter all this virgin territory, the physicists will develop new analytical tools better suited to biological systems. Or maybe on the contrary, their concentration on biology will lead to a change in epistemological aims and an abandonment of the search for universal laws.

We are going down to deeper and deeper levels of knowledge that describe mankind more and more accurately and precisely, and we are approaching the deepest level, the very foundations. But does this lowest level really exist? Isn't it like numbers? For example, if we look at a set of positive real numbers, there is no smallest number in that set. Beyond the one that seems infinitely small, there is always an even smaller one waiting. It may be similar with the hierarchies of knowledge. We are doomed to keep descending into the depths, but we will never be sure we have reached the limits, because there may not be any.

When I was a student, the proton was regarded as the elementary particle. Then quarks were discovered, and in comparison the proton became a complex structure. Some people suspect that even the electron is composite. So is matter infinitely divisible? Will we keep on finding smaller and smaller particles, more and more elementary, because there is no limit where the division stops? Maybe the elements that form the fabric of the world are not particles, but are like strings. Multidimensional space at the deepest level would contain nothing but taut membranes — quantum fields. Vibrating continually and breaking the symmetry, they would emit particles and rays. Each field would send out its own vibrations and the universe would be one super-rich polyphony. It would resound, if not with Plato's "harmony of celestial spheres," then with the modern "quantum canticle."

From behind these elevated concepts that lie beyond the reach of everyday intuition peeps Greek thought. The Greeks consolidated their enchantment with the order and harmony prevailing in nature by extending the expression *kósmos* to mean the entire universe. The word *kósmos* originally meant "beautiful," or "decorative," evidence of which remains in the word "cosmetics." The Greeks noticed this unusual harmony in the construction of living organisms, and they sensed that "the world was an organism rather than anything else." What is the *arché* of the world? they asked. And so they instilled in research into nature the instinct to look for the source, the beginning, the very first principles. The physicians' dreams of a single, unifying theory, with a hidden equation at the very bottom of mankind, are an echo of those dreams. Just like the dreams of modern physicists about the theory of everything, in other words, a theory that focuses all the basic laws about the forces of nature in a sequence of equations. Though the majority regard them as a utopia, these dreams live on. This reverie about the ultimate theory returns like an echo in John Donne's words:

> *If ever any beauty I did see,*
> *Which I desired, and got, 'twas but a dream of thee.*

In the sphere of music, in a sense, Richard Wagner came close to a unifying theory with his idea of a *Gesamtkunstwerk*. In his work music grew out of poetry, and the two of them found their combination in the theater. Thus a space was created where the performers and the audience were united. And Bayreuth—endlessly permeated with music, the gravitation of leading tones and chromatic harmony to an unprecedented degree—was his *Gesamtkunstwerk* come true.

From the dawn of philosophical thought, the question of whether we can understand the world by breaking it down into its elemental parts has been the subject of heated debate. Various answers have been provided, but it is hard to deny that the flourish of the natural sciences is closely connected with reductionism. The tempestuous development that began with the introduction by Galileo of the isolated system continues to this day. Just as in physics and chemistry, reductionism has contributed to the phenomenal development of biology and medicine, reflected in the number of clinical specialties. A hundred years ago neurology and dermatology had already begun to emerge from internal medicine, the queen of medical sciences, and half a century ago cardiology, gastrology, nephrology and many others budded forth. When I was a student, my professors and lecturers used to say proudly: "I am an internist," or "I am a surgeon," and they not only examined the patient, but (after an eventual case conference), they were not afraid to undertake his treatment. Nowadays, if a patient with knee pain applies to the family doctor, he does not even tell him to roll up his trouser leg, but sends him to an orthopedist, who sends him to a rheumatologist, who in his turn sends him to a physiotherapist, etc. Although a narrow specialty is necessary, especially at the university level, it should not obscure a thorough look at the whole of the patient's problems.

Only recently did doubt appear as to whether reductionism was approaching the limits of its potential, because it is an excellent way to research linear reactions. Meanwhile, in the realm of scientific interests dynamic, highly complex, self-organizing systems are appearing. We are perceiving them in the theory of evolution, chaos theory and quantum mechanics, in synergistic effects (which are indeed frequent in medicine), and in the growing field of systems biology. They slip through the net of concepts in which we try to catch them, and dodge out of the way before being trapped in mathematical algorithms. Their components — so abundant that they are hard to count — are internally linked in a non-linear way. Reductionism fails to describe them. We are starting to look for principles that would raise us up, from the deep levels of knowledge we have already achieved to a point where we can embrace the whole, which is something more than the sum of the individual elements. The movement is changing direction, turning back the opposite way. We are talking about "emergence" and looking out for the principles of non-linear thermodynamics, known as "the physics of creative processes." The conviction is spreading and taking root that only non-linear equations can describe the birth of novelties, comprehend and perceive the structures of a whole that is richer than the sum of its parts. Will this really be possible? Let us not forget Democritus's warning: "Do not try to understand everything, because you will find everything incomprehensible." And there is a lot of truth in the tongue-in-cheek remark that natural scientists — physicists, chemists and biologists — work effectively by day as reductionists, and "by night they devote themselves to dreaming about the theory of everything."

The staggering achievements of medicine are inarguably the result of its metamorphosis into a science, enclosing biological research in the rigors that apply to the exact sciences. Even in purely clinical departments where it would seem especially difficult, "evidence-based medicine" is flourishing. Ways of testing drugs in the hospital and of evaluating their efficacy have been strictly established, while also preserving objectivity and impartiality. These standards have been extended to other forms of treatment too, including surgery, rehabilitation, etc. The test results are subjected to severe, critical analysis by groups of specialists, even entire institutes recruited for this purpose, and ultimately — once consensus has been achieved — proclaimed to be recommended standards, principles for medical procedure. Increasingly often, they have the adjective "global" in their name, implying an ambition to cover all the countries in the world. They are regularly amended, and have unquestionably contributed to a crucial rise in the standards of medicine. Some people are offended by their schematism, especially clinicians with a flair for science, though they are not in fact principally aimed at them. Among them we find some rather drastic opinions, such as: "There is no such thing as consensus science. If it's consensus, it isn't science. If it's science, it isn't consensus. Period." Of course, standards, recommendations and consensus all collapse in ruins the moment there is a breakthrough discovery, as happened recently in gastrology.

In the late 1970s Robert Warren, a pathologist at the University of Perth in Australia, working independently, noticed the presence of tiny, curved bacteria in the stomachs of deceased patients. Where there were most of them, the mucous membrane showed features of inflammation. Warren involved a young doctor called Barry Marshall in his research. After laborious attempts they succeeded in cultivating the bacteria in the laboratory. They christened it *Helicobacter pylori*.

No one wanted to believe them. How could bacteria live in the most unfriendly place in our bodies, full of a water solution of hydrochloric acid (pH 1.0–2.0) and digestive enzymes? They gathered a lot of proof, including evidence that *Helicobacter* is the cause of ulcers. But the reviewers were extremely critical. *The Lancet* and other journals refused to accept their work for publication. At this point, after an initial gastroscopy that showed he had a healthy stomach, Marshall drank a small glass of freshly cultivated bacteria. His stomach ached, he felt dizzy, he vomited and his breath smelled "like a sewer." A gastroscopy showed inflammation and ulceration, which was cured with antibiotics. Then *The Lancet* accepted the work for publication, and in 2005 the two scholars won the Nobel Prize for discovering the cause of stomach and duodenal ulcers, as well as a new, effective way of treating them. It is worth adding that *Helicobacter* has been close to us since the dawn of time. When our ancestors emigrated from Africa, they already carried these bacteria inside them. Like a hitchhiker it has moved about with us for at least sixty thousand years.

The blindness of *The Lancet* can be explained by exaggerated caution. Is it really exaggerated? Indeed, not so long ago the world was gazing in admiration at the Korean scientist Hwang Woo-suk. But after being published in the top scientific journals, the results of his research on how we can obtain stem cells from the cloned cells of human embryos turned out to have been faked, entirely fabricated. At roughly the same time an article appeared in *The Lancet* from Oslo about a new potential treatment for cancer of the mouth. It described observations made by studying nine hundred patients, and proved entirely fictitious. The lead author admitted fakery. What role his thirteen co-authors played, including his own twin brother, we can only guess. But let us take pity on *The Lancet* and stop listing its disastrous errors at that.

The more prestigious the journal, the finer the sieve of reviewers through which a paper must force its way before it appears in print. Harsh reviewers feel safe because they are protected by anonymity. Yet they do make some incredible mistakes. One of these involved the story of Jacques Benveniste. When I first met him, towards the end of my studies, he had already had a racing accident, but he enthusiastically encouraged me to drop medicine and take up motor racing. Some fifteen years later he was head of a laboratory at the Pasteur Institute in Paris. Brilliant and charismatic, by then he had the discovery of the platelet-activating factor to his name. One day I was extremely surprised to read a work of his in *Nature*, the leading scientific journal, about "water memory." He claimed that water serving as a solvent preserves a memory of the substances that have reacted in it. The memory continued to last when all trace of the reacting substances had long since gone, and the water itself had been diluted so much that no more than a droplet of the original solution could have remained. The U.S. National Institutes of Health sent three investigators to Paris, specialists in relentlessly tracking down scientific fraud. But they failed to repeat their usual experience at Benveniste's laboratory. He himself spent many long years conducting a debate on the pages of the journals in his efforts to obtain proof of "water memory."

A similar verification of research took place three hundred years ago. In the archives of the Royal Society in London, a fierce debate has been preserved in the form of correspondence between one of the Society's first members — Hevelius, the famous Polish astronomer from Danzig — and a member of the Society's board — Robert Hooke, the brilliant experimenter who was the first person to see cells under a microscope. Hooke had tried to prove that Hevelius's astronomical observations could not be precise, because he did not use a telescope equipped with sights or a micrometer. To settle the dispute, Edmund Halley was sent from London to Danzig; one of the youngest members in the history of the Society, he was the man whose name was later given to the famous comet. After two months of testing Hevelius's observations in minute detail, Halley confirmed their reliability. And so the finest atlas of the sky in Europe, one copy of which Hevelius gave to the king of Poland, Jan III Sobieski, and another to the king of France, Louis XIV, was genuine. No documents have been preserved at the Royal Society showing how Hooke reacted to "the verdict confirming that his adversary was right."

Nowadays, expenditure on scientific research in biology and medicine is reaching astronomical sums and the armies of scientists are growing in arithmetical progression. Apart from the brilliant exceptions, how can we tell who is who among the masses of "scientific workers" out there? Who should be given grants for their research, and who should be promoted? In short, how do we measure recognition in science? How to weigh up success is the question on everybody's lips. In the global village everyone bares all in the search for applause. If you cannot hear the bravos you might as well not be alive at all. Here is what the Polish poet Cyprian Norwid wrote about it:

> *These days success is an idol — he has spread wide*
> *His sorcery like a map of planet Earth;*
> *Even ancient victory has now stepped aside,*
> *In spite of her eternal worth!*

A hundred years ago David Hilbert set the criterion for excellence for a scientific work. It is proportional to the number of works that have been rendered completely irrelevant, or that can be skipped as a result of this new, outstanding work appearing. Thus it creates a higher standard for examining a scientific issue. Theoretical physicists look forward to this sort of work. The brilliant physicist Andrzej Staruszkiewicz writes as follows about the Copenhagen interpretation of quantum physics: "Here we have a real intellectual logjam that has worn everybody out and has had a disastrous effect on the whole of theoretical physics, which has lost its ontological clarity of world vision; anyone who contributes to removing this logjam will be doing humanity a great service."

For several decades the measure of success has been the response, the publicity that a scientific publication receives. It can be counted up and presented numerically as the number of citations gained, in other words, how often a given publication has been cited in the professional journals, especially the most prestigious ones. A whole new trend is developing called bibliometry, or scientometry. Comparing the frequency of citations by authors in various fields of science is risky; the so-called "h" for Hirsch index, which was introduced in 2005 and rapidly gained popularity, was designed to streamline them. But even within the scope of this field itself, doubts can exist. How are we to take the words of the great contemporary mathematician, winner of the 1998 Fields Medal (the equivalent of the Nobel Prize in mathematics), Timothy Gowers, who declared: "Most mathematical publications are incomprehensible to most mathematicians"?

The huge popularity of the citations index can be explained by the fact that it appeals to a major feature of human nature—vanity. "Vanity," wrote Blaise Pascal, "is so anchored in the heart of man that a soldier, a soldier's servant, a cook, a porter brags and wishes to have his admirers. Even philosophers wish for them. Those who write against it want to have the glory of having written well; and those who read it desire the glory of having read it. I who write this have perhaps this desire, and perhaps those who read it . . ." With the radicalism typical of his thinking, Pascal suggested that scientific works should be published anonymously, without giving the author's name, cutting them off from the anticipation of applause, from vanity and all-embellishing *amour propre*. One of his contemporaries made the following comment on his proposal: "It's easy for him to speak. If he publishes a work anonymously, even so everyone in Europe will know who it is by!"

Zbigniew Herbert's words sound like an echo of Pascal:

> *The Old Masters*
> *did without names.*
> *their signatures were*
> *the white fingers of the Madonna*

Let us leave the index of citations in peace, although it would be a very good thing in Poland if the ministries, universities and scientific institutes chose to make regular use of it in assigning research grants. But let us try to find other ways of measuring the value of scientific work. Nothing is better than time, that is for sure. Time separates the wheat from the chaff. But we refuse to wait, we simply cannot, because we won't be here any more when the truth is revealed. We want it all here and now. However, there are no recipes for scientific discovery or for success. Max Delbrück, a brilliant physicist who introduced scientific thought, analytical and quantitative, to biology, reckoned that in performing an experiment we should admit a certain degree of freedom, some flexibility, in order to perceive the unexpected, the surprise that is worth far more than the expected result. He called this "the principle of limited sloppiness." The British and the Americans use the word "serendipity," a lucky hit, an unexpected discovery, which does not mean an accidental one at all. That was how Ryszard Gryglewski discovered prostacyclin. Professor John Vane had given him a sample of unstable chemical compounds (professionally called endoperoxides PGG^2 and PGH^2) to investigate in which organs (and whether at all) they produce thromboxane A^2, a substance that had just been discovered in the small blood cells, thrombocytes. So, with varied results, Gryglewski tested ground-up cells (homogenates) from various animal organs. When he added the test compounds to some arterial homogenates (microsomes of the aorta), thromboxane was not produced and nothing happened. Most of us would have regarded that as a negative result and moved on. But he noticed that even so, there were less of the added compounds. Could they have changed into something else? He sought the advice of chemists and looked in various books, but he couldn't find the answer. Then he had a brilliant thought. Maybe something so volatile was produced that it immediately dissolved at room temperature? So he set a trap for that "something" by repeating the experiment on ice. This time the detector system showed the appearance of something that was unknown. It was prostacyclin. In the British laboratory where we were working, at first no one wanted to believe in this "Polish hormone which sort of is, but isn't," as they called it. In a series of quick, ingenious experiments Gryglewski and his colleagues provided proof of the existence of prostacyclin—an important natural defensive substance that protects our arteries. Its effect on the human system was then defined and introduced into therapy here in Krakow.

Intuition helps us to sense reality, as it were, to guess at it, or even see it. We value it highly, though it eludes definition.

The word has its origins in the Latin *intueri*, meaning "to examine." It is this intuitive flash of the subconscious, this "short-cut around reason" that sometimes lets the doctor see what is going on in the patient's body. We experience a sort of inner revelation, an insight into the heart of the matter, into things that had seemed hidden from sight . . . Looking at my own everyday medical work, I am sure I do not devote a lot of time to thought, like a mathematician or a physicist. No—medical practice is not just a rational act. As I listen to the history of the illness, as I make observations, perform tests, make my diagnosis and implement treatment, I feel like an elk moving through a forest it knows pretty well: it catches scents and sounds, and looks for clues . . . It tracks these impressions and uses them to build up a picture that will enable it to react as precisely as possible. There is often something that makes me wonder, because it diverges from the norm and doesn't form a familiar shape. Then the mystery works away inside me, only to come back unexpectedly at night, or a few days later, sometimes again and again, with a solution that may not be right at all.

And as for rationalism . . . One morning I am on my daily ward round. I enter a ward where a forty-year-old female patient is lying in bed. She complains of sleeping badly—she cannot get to sleep before four AM. "Then I read your book, *Catharsis*," she says. "Aha, and it sends you to sleep," I say. "No, it doesn't," the embarrassed patient tries to defend herself. "Maybe it's this pillow that's stopping you from sleeping?" She is lying on a pillow embroidered with a drawing by Polish satirical cartoonist Andrzej Mleczko, showing the devil tempting a woman. The patient looks at me incredulously.

A week later I come to see her again, in the same bed, in the same ward. "I'm sleeping well now," she says. "I changed my pillow."

When a new scientific discovery is made, we see something no one has ever seen before us, sometimes that no one has even imagined might exist. Whereas in clinical practice there are times when we dream of noticing something we have already seen before. This happens when days or even weeks go by, but the scattered symptoms of an illness refuse to form a pattern, we cannot make a diagnosis and we do not know what is wrong with the patient. But maybe we have seen it before? Isn't it a repeat, a rerun, but of what?

When my younger son reached the age of five, he started taking an interest in everything I was doing. One evening I was working on a lecture. He wanted me to tell him about it. "It's a good thing, that sort of lecture," he said once he had heard me out. "You put it together once, and then you keep repeating it to the students every year." "I never repeat myself!" I replied indignantly. Next day he came up to me with a clean sheet of paper. "Sign here, please." I signed. Then from behind his back he pulled out my ID card and showed me the signatures, on the card and on the sheet of paper. They were identical. Then he asked triumphantly: "So you never repeat yourself?"

So it is as if the doctor uses one hemisphere of the brain—the creative one—to seek new solutions, while using the other to watch out for repetitions. And so he develops his art, his skills. When we talk of first-rate skills, of the heights of the medical art, we think of the virtuosity of a surgeon. Comparing him with a virtuoso pianist or violinist does not seem far off the mark. And just as in music, this excellence sometimes has family roots in surgery too. Alexis Carrel is a good example. He developed vascular surgery, creating the foundations for organ transplants. His work was crowned with the Nobel Prize for medicine in 1912, the first time it had been awarded to a scientist working in the United States. Operating on the blood vessels is a fine art. To prick small arteries without causing bleeding and then join their ends together, with a straight stitch and diagonally, pulling the thread gently but firmly — all this demands exceptional dexterity. And what if the operating field shrinks, as we operate on small creatures — mice, guinea pigs, or . . . babies? It is as intricate as making lace. Alexis Carrel, a Frenchman who emigrated to the United States, learned this art from the lacemakers of Lyons, one of whom was his mother.

Watching a brilliant surgeon at work, actively participating in an operation, can be a kind of aesthetic experience. There is not a single superfluous movement, just fluency, confidence and rhythm. This rhythm takes over the entire company, and the whole team starts to move as if in a trance. It looks as if they could close their eyes and the operation would keep going on its own. But if an unforeseen obstacle arises, followed at once by another, and then yet another — each of which is capable of ruining everything in an instant — you have to face up to them and deal with the unexpected. The surgeon must have the presence of mind to take a leap into the dark, a split-second decision. Whether or not to jump into deep water — like the question that suddenly confronted Lord Jim in Joseph Conrad's novel and the narrator in Albert Camus's *The Fall*. "Because the summit of surgery," as a talented young cardiac surgeon once told me, "is not achieved by phenomenal dexterity." On the summit, as at Wimbledon, we find the very best players.

Each of them hits the ball perfectly and knows all the tricks of tennis. But the one who is master of the situation wins. He never loses his head, he never gets lost and he never lets himself get confused. He sees the inevitability and irreversibility of the situation created by his movements, and controls the field of play. He is like a sculptor who aims to extract a figure from a block of marble, but knows that one wrong move of the hammer and chisel will write off the entire operation.

There was a time, about two hundred years ago, when science and art were woven together in biology by thick threads, natural observations and speculations that were sometimes hard to distinguish. This rich conglomerate produced Goethe's and the German Romantics' *Naturphilosophie*. They were fascinated by the profound, mysterious similarity between forms of Nature that lay hidden within its diversity. To explain the shapes and morphic features repeated in countless variants, they coined the concept of the archetype. And they examined the archetype, this "conception of Nature," in its transformations and metamorphoses, uniting poet and scholar, and both of them with Nature. Darwinism put an end to this philosophy of Nature, although Darwin himself was a great admirer of Humboldt, who advocated *Naturphilosophie* and was a friend of Goethe. Humboldt was convinced there were patterns, basic forms concealed behind the richness of the world of plants. He sought them out, brought them to light and even defined their number as sixteen. For him they were like recurring musical themes, in which the species and families of plants played the variations. Alexander von Humboldt — traveler, romantic adventurer, author of a powerful synthesis of natural history knowledge about the Earth and the universe — preceded Darwin on a scientific voyage to the sub-equatorial countries of South America, a voyage that also took him five years. Darwin read his famous diaries from the voyage when he was still a student at Cambridge. He took the first two volumes with him on the *Beagle*. In his notes from the expedition he wrote: "I am at present fit only to read Humboldt; he like another Sun illumines everything I behold." And years later he added: "I never forget that my whole course of life is due to having read and reread as a Youth his Personal Narrative." He remained enchanted by Humboldt's prose and shared his delight in Nature. He unconsciously imitated his style to such an extent that his sister Caroline pointed it out to him: "you have without perceiving it got to embody your ideas in his poetical language." It is worth remembering this Darwin — sensitive, romantic and passionate. How different he is from the image history has handed down to us, in the widely distributed posthumous portrait, from which a venerable old man glares at us like a terrifying Old Testament prophet.

A hundred years later, the "philosophy of Nature" came back like an echo in the work of Ernst Haeckel, a professor of zoology in Jena who was an oceanographer. Haeckel had wanted to be a landscape painter, but he became obsessed with sea creatures. He spent twelve years studying amoebae, documenting four thousand species of them, a truly astounding number. He made no plans to write a manual based on his own scientific research, but presented his discoveries in the form of art. He was fascinated by the mysterious forms of Nature, including those that are only visible under a microscope, and devoted hundreds of drawings to them. He drew and painted in color, decoratively, in Art Nouveau style, and in 1904 he published a work entitled *Kunstformen der Natur* ("The Shapes of Art in Nature"), which delighted all Europe. Amid a wealth of shapes and colors, our vision is usually drawn to the centrally positioned specimen, from which the other varieties radiate in the shape of a fan. It is the core form that contains the essence of the structure. This is "organic crystallography," according to

Haeckel, who reckoned all forms of increasing complexity were derived from a common model. From his illustrations, which are among the very finest ever produced on the topic of nature, order, symmetry and hierarchy shine out. They reveal a logic and a purpose that we would seek in vain within the struggle for existence, within natural selection. Haeckel's famous theory (known as "biogenetic law"), that evolution recurs in the embryonic development of organisms, was an attempt to find a unifying formula within the world of Nature. Nowadays, some people accuse him of lending symmetry to creatures viewed under the microscope as well as with the naked eye, of creating ideal, Platonic beings. "Their very beauty betrays them," they say. As if beauty could not exist within Nature, or outside art.

Even today, when genetics provides us with rational explanations for hidden though striking similarities, we can hear a note that sounded for the first time in Jena. Doesn't evolution converge, doesn't it reach for the same solutions, even in species that are distant from each other? some people ask. And they claim that the convergence of solutions is universal, despite immeasurable genetic possibilities. And so despite an endless number of roads, "life navigates to precise end-points." We should say that these original views are isolated, and as they break free of the standard convictions of the evolutionism, they are criticized for smacking of creationism. Yet something is changing as a result of the most recent discoveries, concerning milk intolerance, for example. In childhood milk is our most important food. But in adulthood most people (except for those of European origin) cease to assimilate lactose, which is the sugar in milk. It happens because the gene that oversees production of the enzyme that breaks lactose down into simple, assimilable components goes quiet and gets switched off. Without it milk and its products are hard to absorb, so they not only cease to taste good to us, they even irritate the alimentary canal. In 2002 a mutation was described among the Finns, which causes this same gene controlling the synthesis of lactose to remain active after childhood, rather than dying out. So adult Finns can consume milk without any trouble. Two years later, among those inhabitants of Kenya and Tanzania who assimilated milk well, the identical "Finnish mutation" could not be found. Yet the same gene as in the Finns had changed and mutated in them too, except that it happened at an adjacent point. And so one single gene underwent various mutations in different parts of the world, resulting in exactly the same effect. This has been recognized as "the best example of convergent evolution in human beings."

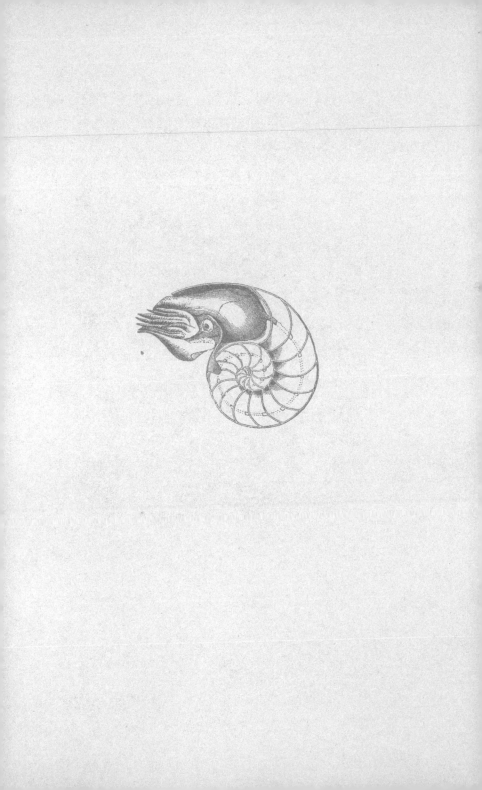

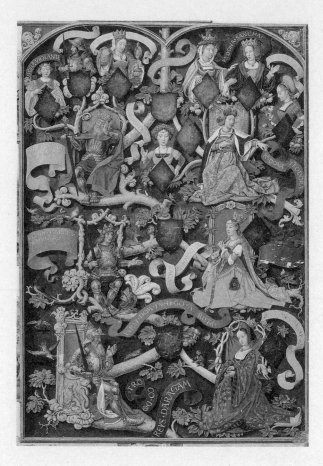

Simon Bening, António de Holanda
The Genealogical Tree of the Kings of Aragon, 1530–1534
British Library, London

GENETICS AND CANCER

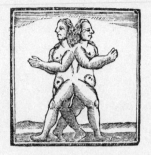

Laetum non omnis finit, or "Death does not end everything," we read on the grave of Joseph Brodsky at San Michele cemetery in the Venice Laguna. Franz Kafka defined death lightheartedly, almost jokingly, as "an apparent end that produces real suffering." Both these comments hint at the idea of an indestructible element, the eternity that a man carries inside him and that does not die with him. Ovid simply called it the soul, for only "souls are all exempt from power of death" (*morte carent animae*). The English poet Thomas Hardy also considered the capacity of physical, bodily features to survive. He saw them recurring from generation to generation—the shape of the eyelids, the line of the lips, a smile, the timbre of a voice—they said "no" to impermanence and conquered time. And in a poem entitled *Heredity* he wrote as follows:

> *I am the family face;*
> *Flesh perishes, I live on,*
> *Projecting trait and trace*
> *Through time to times anon,*

And leaping from place to place
Over oblivion.

One of the most famous genetic features to manifest itself for eighteen generations was the conspicuous protruding lower lip of the Habsburgs. Yet it cannot have deprived the family's princesses of charm, as six of them married Polish kings, from Kazimierz the Jagiellonian to Zygmunt III. They were the personification of the maxim "*Belli gerant alii, tu, felix Austria, nube!*" ("Let others wage war, you, fortunate Austria, marry!"). For centuries marriages extended the hereditary estates of the Habsburgs far and wide, giving them the Netherlands, the Spanish throne, and the crowns of Hungary and the Czech lands.

Hanging on the dining room wall in our apartment is a portrait of my mother in early youth. We had looked at it all our lives without actually seeing it, and certainly without connecting it in any way with my daughter Ania. But when Ania turned fourteen, one day we noticed that she was starting to resemble the portrait. Over the next few days the similarity became striking. The young woman in the portrait and the girl in the room facing her looked like mirror images of each other. So it was for a fortnight, but then they began to draw apart and diverge, like clouds passing over the mountains. And just as it had appeared, the similarity vanished, never to return again.

Charles Darwin explained heredity as follows: each mature organ produces tiny particles, "gemmules," in which its essence is contained. They amass in the reproductive cells and are passed on to the progeny, recreating within it the organs from which they grew. In the early twentieth century, when Thomas Hardy wrote his poem *Heredity*, people were mindful of the experiments conducted by the Moravian monk, Gregor Mendel; by crossing peas in the monastery garden he had discovered the basic laws of genetics. At the same time August Weismann established that we carry two cell lines within us: somatic and embryonic, separate lines between which there has always been a partition. And so he revealed to us an incredible continuum, a continuity that reaches back from every cell living today into the abyss of time and indicates a relationship between us and all living creatures inhabiting the Earth, both in the animal and the plant worlds.

Fifty years later came the discovery of the double helix of DNA, the treasure store of the genetic code, hidden deep within the nucleus of the cell. And in another fifty years, at the start of the current century, the code was deciphered, letter by letter, three billion letters in all, and ... posted on the Internet. This spectacular result, the fruit of the work of hundreds of scientists, concentrated in two rival research groups, has become the symbol of our era, the third millennium. It has been showered in high-flown epithets, which echo with such phrases as "the book of life" and "the Bible of Nature." One Nobel Prize winner even declared: "we will know what it is to be human," to which another one retorted ironically: "We have the sequence now (or most of it, at least), and what we know principally is that we are stunningly similar to chimpanzees in the makeup of our genes."

Fifty-five years after the discovery of the structure of DNA and its publication in the journal *Nature*, James Watson decoded the genome and published the results in the same journal. It was he, together with Francis Crick, who by cutting out pieces of cardboard to make three-dimensional models of DNA, imagined that they are arranged in the shape of a double helix. The fact that the genome was "decoded" by the great Nobel Prize winner has powerful symbolic significance. However, more symbolic than biological, because having a recording of the three billion letters of his

DNA sequence does not even allow us to work out such simple features of Watson as his height, not to mention his predisposition to certain illnesses. Certainly, as time passes we often refer to this publication. But if we want to talk about Watson himself, we will have to rely — in the manner of modern historians — "on what Watson wrote, said and did during his lifetime, rather than on the order of the base pairs in his genome."

At the beginning of 2008 only two people in the world had had their individual genetic sequences decoded (the other person apart from Watson was the American geneticist Craig Venter). It is estimated that at the turn of 2011 and 2012 there were about 30,000 people in this category. The phenomenal rise in their numbers is the result of technological progress. Powerful, ultra-fast sequencers are being introduced, in other words, machines that can read the order of the letters in a genome, known as next-generation sequencing technologies. The price of decoding is falling, and is at present less than ten thousand dollars. And therefore shall we too soon be "decoded," shall we all become the owners of our "personal genetic evidence"? And will medicine take on "personalized" colors? Does this mean that by sequencing our own genome we shall be able to draw conclusions about our susceptibility to particular illnesses, and if we do fall sick, shall we be able to apply "personalized" drugs, in other words, drugs tailored to the individual patient? This vision of the future has many supporters within contemporary medicine.

After the decoding of the genome, doctors and biologists — and in their wake patients and their families — believed we had succeeded in finding within the genome the *loci*, or sites of illnesses, especially some common ones. This would be a specific configuration of genes, perhaps mutant, which would mean a predisposition to the development of frequent multifactor diseases. But this did not happen. The entire genome was thoroughly screened, and associations were sought between certain sections of it and a given illness. It was laborious, lengthy research, involving thousands or even tens of thousands of patients. Certain connections were found between genetic variants and particular illnesses, but their force, the strength of the links, was not great. They did not determine the development of the disease, or enable an earlier diagnosis. These associations build up into more and more complex images of the development of illnesses, but they do not bring any decisive answers. Neither arteriosclerosis, nor in particular coronary disease, neither asthma, rheumatoid arthritis or schizophrenia, Alzheimer's disease or multiple sclerosis—the plagues of modern civilization—revealed their essential secrets (we shall shortly talk of cancers separately). They vary in this respect from rare congenital diseases such as hemophilia, cystic fibrosis or alpha-1 antitrypsin deficiency—in all of which it has been possible to show the mutations of individual genes and their definitive causal connection with the disease.

Nevertheless, in the United States prediction of the risk of common diseases, based on variations in genome (called "single nucleotide polymorphisms," or SNPs) is available on the Internet from over sixty companies. Direct sale of kits in retail stores has been blocked by the FDA, which has taken the view that consumers should only be able to assess clinical genetic tests through a doctor in order to avoid any misunderstanding about the significance of the results. At present, for most conditions "an individual's risk will be changed only slightly by the results of the tests." However, with technology rapidly improving, "an all-inclusive price of $1,000 per genome is soon likely to become a reality." Interpreting anyone's complete genome sequence will be a great challenge, since rare variants seen only in that person will carry uncertain consequences.

♦♦♦

Ten years after the decoding of the genome, it was judged that the clinical repercussions of the discovery were "modest." So has this epoch-making discovery failed to translate into clinical medicine? Hasn't it left its mark on medical practice? Is it different from the other great discoveries? Indeed, after Ernst Chain and Howard Florey described the curative effectiveness of penicillin in 1941, it saved the lives of thousands of people. The same thing happened with hormones of the adrenal cortex, synthesized in 1946. So is it fair to say that transferring the great discovery connected with the decoding of DNA into medical practice will take several generations? This claim seems overly pessimistic. The matter really has proved extraordinarily complicated, and has caused many difficulties and disappointments. Fascinated by the great discovery, we have let ourselves believe that the goal has been reached and the summit climbed, as if the way forward is well mapped out and visible. Meanwhile, science always takes us on a journey where no point that we reach is the end of the line, but just a stop that reveals a road winding on into the unknown. In the case of genetics there have been many surprises in store along that road.

Shortly after the decoding of the genome, it became clear that genes represent at most two percent of DNA, so they were compared to oases scattered among the desert sands. This desert consists of motifs that are repeated tens of thousands of times over. The simplest ones are tandems, built of two letters in the code, for example, GT, GT, . . . , GT. Others are incomparably more complicated. Many of them are mobile and move from place to place, like the shifting sands of the desert. No one knows why we have this desert inside us. The molecular biologists have found themselves in the same situation as the astronomers — for about twenty years they have known that the universe is not nearly as empty as it seems, but is filled with strange "(non-baryonic) matter that is different from ours," and also a mysterious energy. Invisible to our eyes, they are defined by the adjective "black." We conclude that they exist on the basis of their dual effect: on the movement of distant galaxies and on the acceleration of space. The ignorance of the molecular biologists is comparable with the astronomers' ignorance. Just as over ninety-five percent of matter and energy in the universe is "black" and mysterious, so too "desert" DNA remains a mystery, hidden in impenetrable darkness.

This "black" DNA — to use the astronomers' adjective — is often called "junk," in other words, scrap or even garbage. Until recently it did not attract any attention. Who would want to rummage in the garbage? Some sort of molecular vagrant, perhaps? Yet we can assume the number of these vagrants is going to grow fast, because there is treasure hidden in the garbage heap. It might be a storage container for ready-to-use segments for "nature's evolutionary experiments." Consider the duplication of genes, for example. One gene remains unchanged, while the other undergoes a mutation. Does this cause changes in the organism, and of what kind? We would have to wait for a repeat of the same experiment. But if mutant genes of exactly this kind are ready and waiting within the scrap, in easy reach and instantly available for use, the entire process is speeded up. There may also be elements of the highest rank hidden within the scrap heap which regulate the expression of genes.

Transposons are candidates for this specific role. What amazing . . . creatures, I would like to say! Transposons are mobile genetic elements that cut themselves out of the genome of their own accord and move, sometimes a long way, down the thread of DNA, and then inscribe themselves within it again in a different place. They can also jump horizontally, from cell to cell, or even from one species to another, especially among the simplest organisms. "Scissors" (transposases) code themselves, guaranteeing a precise excision in the thread of DNA, and so does "glue," which allows them to re-embed themselves again, sometimes after a very long journey. Sometimes they are called "sailors," because they sail along the genome by themselves, without the complicity or help of other proteins.

In man they form almost half the genome, but only about one percent of them have preserved their mobility and can still jump from point to point. The rest are dormant. On the other hand, in simple organisms, such as bacteria and fruit flies, the percentage of these active elements is much higher. Presumably, transposons were the motor of evolution. Indeed, their wanderings about the genome are not neutral. By inscribing themselves in a new region of the DNA, they caused the genes to mutate or the chromosomes to be rearranged, and if these features were advantageous to the host, they were retained in succeeding generations. Once they had colonized vertebrates, the transposons were rendered inactive, put to sleep. Yet this one percent in man, the one that is not dormant, may be the cause of illnesses. And so it is suspected that hemophilia, Duchenne muscular dystrophy and cancers—of the esophagus as well as the nipple and ovaries—"might develop as a result of SINE or LINE inscribing themselves in certain genes or their close neighborhood." These abbreviations stand for categories of transposons; for example, the genome of each of us contains about half a million copies of LINE ("long interspersed nuclear elements"), of which from fifty to a hundred are still mobile, capable of moving.

The gene first emerged as an idea, to materialize years later. It is still with us, though sometimes we start wondering whether we shouldn't send it back into the world of ideas. It was first heard of in 1909, from the lips of a Danish botanist called Wilhelm Johannsen, who coined the name "gene" for a hypothetical element conditioning an innate feature. Soon after, scientists discovered, in fruit flies, that chromosomes determine inheritance, and they imagined that genes are inherent within them, like beads strung on a thread. The next fact to be accepted was that they are built of DNA, whose structure was discovered in 1953 by James Watson and Francis Crick. Inheritance can be summarized in shorthand as follows: an organism has the instructions for how to create its successor enclosed within the capsules of the gametes. These instructions are passed on to the fertilized egg cell and gradually reveal themselves within it, until a descendant comes into being. The instructions are in the shape of the double DNA thread, are located in the chromosomes and are written in a four-letter code that defines the shape of the organism and all its functions. Individual sentences from these instructions are rewritten as orders, which are carried by special envoys — called mRNA, where "m" is for messenger — from the nucleus of the cell to the cytoplasm, where proteins are formed out of amino acids. The flow of information is transparent and in one direction: from DNA to RNA and onwards — to the site of protein synthesis. The assignment is unambiguous: one gene creates one enzyme (one protein).

In recent years this lucid pattern, known as the central dogma of molecular biology, has started to be filled with such a wealth of unexpected details that at times it looks as if its central line is becoming obliterated. Let us mention at least three discoveries that have shaken it to its foundations. Firstly, each gene is built of a few to about a dozen blocks, which can be put together in various configurations during their conversion, their "rewriting" into mRNA. And so from one gene various amino acids and proteins can arise. The unambiguity of the instructions — within the thread of DNA — gets blurred. Secondly, there is no rule saying that the activated messengers (mRNA) will reach their destination with the message. On the contrary, many of them will go quiet before setting off on the journey, because the DNA thread will send short segments after them, called micro-RNA, which will lock onto them and silence them. Thirdly, mRNA can not just be messengers carrying instructions passed down from above, but can also carry messages in themselves that they hand on from generation to generation, without the involvement of headquarters, i.e., the DNA. And finally, there are the genes themselves. We are ceasing to regard them as closed, limited units of inheritance, even if they are made up of small blocks inside. They do not seem to have a start or end, they overlap over extensive areas and we cannot see their limits because they form a continuum. These views are reflected in the definition of a gene recently proposed by twenty-five eminent specialists: "a locatable region of genomic sequence, corresponding to a unit of inheritance, which is associated with regulatory regions, transcribed regions and/or other functional sequence regions." We have come a long way from the simple definition of a gene from almost a hundred years ago.

The primitive aborigines of New Guinea have contributed to undermining the accepted laws of genetics. They have a custom of eating the brain of a dead relative at the wake, which causes them to contract a dangerous neuro-degenerative disease called "kuru." The disease is triggered by particular proteins, called "prions." They are also the cause of mad cow disease and scrapie in sheep. Prions do not contain nucleic acids; they are neither DNA nor RNA. Thus they are different from all previously known infectious factors — bacteria and viruses. Yet they are carriers of information, and are able to pass this information on to the cells. They belong to the elements of inheritance that are not subject to Mendel's laws. They operate by changing the recipient's spatial structure. And so one prion protein can affect another, causing a change in its conformation (in other words its three-dimensional, spatial shape), and this change is then passed on to other proteins. This new mechanism regulates the activity of some enzymes and cooperates in the creation of long-term memory. However, it does not seem to play a role in the development of cancers.

Among the modern breakthrough discoveries in genetics on which doctors are pinning particular hopes are the small particles of RNA known as micro-RNA. It was for them that in 2006 Andrew Z. Fire and Craig C. Mello won the Nobel Prize. They develop within the DNA in a natural way, but we already know how to synthesize them in a test tube. With the help of micro-RNA we can switch off individual genes, changing the flow of genetic information. Until now, such possibilities were limited. At one end of the information flow we have corticosteroids at our disposal (natural or synthetic hormones of the adrenal cortex). However, their action is not selective. They shape the transcription process (the "rewriting" of RNA from DNA), suppressing some genes while stimulating others. At the other end of the information chain, in other words, the translation of mRNA into polypeptides (the start of protein synthesis), the intervention possibilities have already been exploited to a large degree. So, for example, antibiotics suppress the translation of bacterial ribosomes, which fortunately are different from human ones.

Perhaps in about a dozen years we will have drugs at our disposal that work by using micro-RNA to silence genes. Given to the patient, they would block the expression of proteins that cause incurable illnesses. There are many genes whose silencing could bring therapeutic benefits. The problem is that although micro-RNA are so small, as their name emphasizes, they arouse the organism's defensive immune response, which in this case is undesirable. Several ingenious strategies have already been devised to bypass this defense. Preliminary, cautious clinical tests were undertaken in 2007 in two illnesses where topical application is advisable. These are macular degeneration (direct injection into the vitreous body of the eye) and respiratory syncytial virus, an infection that is common in children (application by nasal spray).

When asked if cancer is hereditary, we reply — usually with relief — "But of course not!" Naturally, we may have heard of some unusual family blighted with cancer, and physicians have a lively interest in this sort of family. But those are rather exceptional cases. It is also possible, though it happens extremely rarely, for a pregnant woman suffering from a cancer to pass the illness on to her fetus (e.g., leukemia, melanoma). In these cases, however, the cancer cells pervade the fetus directly through the placenta. So can we be sure cancer has nothing to do with genetics? The most important achievement in oncology in the past few decades has been to prove the falsity of this claim and to demonstrate beyond all doubt that cancers do originate within the genes — in altered, mutant genes. In the substantial majority of cases they are somatic mutations; in other words, they occurred during the individual life, and do not involve the embryonic line, so they are not passed on to descendants.

Many factors cause cancerous mutations of the DNA. They pervade us by various routes from the surrounding world. As early as 1761, one London doctor conjectured that taking snuff caused nasal cancer to develop. Fourteen years later, his colleague Percival Pitt, who has gone down in the annals of medicine for all time, noticed the frequent appearance of cancer of the perineum in British chimney sweeps and ascribed it to contact with soot, which contains not fully burned carbon residues. With the dawning of the Industrial Revolution, and then the technological one in the twentieth century, these first observations, which nowadays we would call epidemiological, were increased by the addition of coal dust, asbestos, aniline dyes and many others. In the early 1950s the first observations were published in the United States indicating that in habitual smokers the likelihood of developing lung cancer is forty times higher. Half a year later they were confirmed in Britain, and so began the crusade against smoking that is still going on today.

Scientists needed an experimental model for prompting cancer. In 1915 it was provided by two Japanese, who discovered that all you had to do was to rub tar into the ear of a rabbit. They were lucky in choosing a species of animal that is particularly sensitive to this carcinogen as well as the right spot to apply it. But they also proved commendable for persistence in their research. To trigger the cancer, they regularly smeared the tar in exactly the same spot, every other day for one hundred days. In his elation after making the discovery, one of the two experimenters, Katsusaburo Yamagiwa, wrote a haiku in superb calligraphy: "I have made cancer. / I have proudly proceeded / several steps forward." History judged that he had a legitimate reason to be proud, because he showed the way forward towards identifying carcinogens and proved that tumors develop as a result of events that are repeated many times over.

The history of breakthrough research in cancer abounds in unusual characters. Let us offer three examples. In 1903, twenty-five-year-old Walter Sutton, a medical student at Columbia University, published a paper entitled "The Chromosomes in Heredity." While keenly researching grasshoppers, he came to conclusions that are nowadays at the core of biology teaching in every high school: 1) all multicellular organisms contain double sets of distinctive chromosomes; 2) as a result of division, descendant cells receive one chromosome from the father and one from the mother; and 3) sperm and egg cells get only one chromosome each, but this number doubles after fertilization. On the basis of these observations, he realized that chromosomes are the carriers of hereditary traits, and this breakthrough discovery puts him on a par with Mendel and Watson and Crick. Sutton created the entire science of cytogenetics and identified the genetic system of cells. All this in one student publication, because he never published another. He gave up scientific research in favor of surgery, and died young, at the age of thirty-nine.

A quarter of a century after him, a Texan named Hermann Joseph Muller discovered that X-rays, a recognized carcinogen, cause mutation of the genes in fruit flies (*Drosophila melanogaster*). But this time there was no haiku — quite the opposite. The forty-one-year-old American's work was given an extremely critical reception that, combined with a difficult period in his marriage, drove him to depression. Without much delay, he took a large dose of sleeping pills and wandered into the woods outside the city of Austin. Like many other suicides, he had a note on him, which read: "My period of usefulness, if I had one, now seems about over." Alarmed by his disappearance, his colleagues frantically began to comb the woods together, and next day they found him, in a coma, but alive. Fifteen years later, in 1946, Muller won the Nobel Prize for the discovery of experimental mutagenesis.

And finally, a visionary called Theodor Boveri, who was a professor of biology at the University of Würzburg. In his first papers he had already offered the conjecture that cancer might be caused by damage to or a lack of chromosomes in the cell. It is not entirely clear where he got this idea from, as he had not been researching cancerous chromosomes. His work went unnoticed, but he continued his idea and developed it fully in a book published in 1914, entitled *The Origin of Malignant Tumors* (*Zur Frage der*

Entstehung maligner Tumoren), whose significance for biology and medicine has been compared to that of Newton's *Principia* for classical physics. The book's main thesis went: "The unrestrained tendency of cancer cells towards rapid proliferation may arise from the domination of the chromosomes that promote cell division. Another explanation for cancer is the presence of defined chromosomes that suppress cell division. Cancer cells would set off on the path of development if these restraining chromosomes were eliminated." For modern biologists, geneticists and oncologists, these are "landmark conclusions" whose accuracy was confirmed over half a century later.

For nowadays we know that every human tumor that has been thoroughly examined is a combination of changes in two types of genes: proto-oncogenic and suppressor genes. They work in opposite ways. If the molecular reactions that control the life of a cell can be compared to a network of complex electrical circuits, there are two kinds of commutators within it. Stimulating one kind leads to a short circuit that, by keeping going, violently accelerates the flow of current (reaction). This is what the mutation of proto-oncogenes involves. The second kind are brakes that slow down the circulation. Eliminating them removes the brakes, and the current (reaction), now free of obstacles, takes on unusual speed.

The vast number of mutations is staggering. When the entire genetic record of a cancer cell from a lung cancer patient was read, 22,910 somatically acquired substitutions were identified in the genetic code (somatic mutations), while in another patient with a malignant melanoma, this number totaled 33,345. Yet this includes the disappearance of entire blocks of the recording (deletions) or the unexpected inclusion of new "words" (insertions). In this panorama, it is no longer possible to speak of any kind of harmony of cells. The mutated genes blow up the tissue with their primitive energy, ultimately leading to the destruction of the organism.

◆◆◆

These staggering discoveries in the field of the molecular biology of cancers that are revealing to us their origin and development have not yet found their reflection in therapy. Mortality because of cancer is today almost the same as it was fifty years ago (though in 2006 it showed a small downward trend for the first time), whereas mortality because of heart diseases, cerebrovascular diseases and infectious diseases has decreased by nearly two-thirds! The brilliant oncologist Harold Varmus reckons that surgery, chemotherapy and radiotherapy will remain the basis of cancer treatment for many years to come. They are becoming increasingly effective thanks to a technological revolution. It is all to do with aiming the drugs or radioactivity straight at the cancer without disturbing the surrounding area. So, for example, by using radioactive implants we are able to bombard the tumor directly, without touching the organs next to it. And what if we were to remove a healthy, delicate organ from the neighborhood of a tumor, an organ that would certainly be irreversibly damaged by the planned treatment, preserve it outside the system during the treatment, and once it was over, implant it back in its place? This actually happened in France recently, where a young woman suffering from cancer of the lymphatic system was obliged to undergo a draconian course of treatment, using radioactivity and drugs. There was no doubt at all that the proposed therapy would have destroyed her ovaries. So they were removed from her body and placed in liquid nitrogen at a temperature of minus one hundred and ninety-seven degrees Celsius. Then she underwent the treatment, which lasted for months on end but proved successful. At this point the patient's ovaries were re-implanted in her abdominal cavity. The thirty-two-year-old woman became pregnant, and — cured of her cancer — gave birth to a healthy child!

However, the results are not always so extraordinary. Sometimes oncological treatment is cut short because each new stage brings more suffering, or it is too late, and the tumor can no longer be cured. There is no textbook standard here, no stop sign. Where should we look for it? "In experience, understood as the memory of errors made." This is what tells us when to take a risk or even to act in defiance of the accepted protocol, and when to abandon treatment. Another invaluable element is the patient's own determination, his desire to fight the cancer, which the doctor can influence.

Conventional therapies, whether using chemical drugs, radioactivity, or surgery, aim to destroy the cancer cells, or at least limit their development. But they do not get to the source of the cancer; they do not try to attack or eradicate its cause. This sort of effective, causal action has only been undertaken in recent years, and that at the molecular level. It involves using drugs to intervene into the network of intercellular signals. What sort of a network is it? On the surface of the cell, in the membrane surrounding it, there are docking places, fastening points, for very many chemical substances, such as hormones or drugs. The chemical substances flow in from the bloodstream, or via the lymph or nerves, or develop locally. They anchor in the cell membrane in these "docks" that are specially prepared for them called receptors. The impetus of their "docking" releases a signal that travels from the surface of the cell to the nucleus, where it arouses selected genes within the DNA. However, it does not take a direct route. The signal is passed on by specific chemical molecules that create a sort of chain of transmitters. These "chains," the paths along which the signals travel, are extremely numerous. They intersect and merge together; in short, they create a virtual network—a network of intercellular signals. Sometimes an individual transmitter, a component within the extremely complex chain, is faulty because an error, a mutation, has developed in its DNA recording. In chronic myeloid leukemia the error is so dense that it can be seen under a microscope as a shortening of one of the chromosomes, which has been given the name *Philadelphia*. As a result, a faulty transmitter protein is formed that places itself at the very beginning of the chain of transmitters. It causes violent and permanent acceleration of transmission along several paths. The signals bombard the cell nucleus, which goes into overproduction of white blood cells in the bone marrow. The crazy transmitter can be suppressed, and the drug that can do it is called imatinib. It was introduced into therapy in the twenty-first century, ever since the fates of patients with a relatively common form of leukemia have changed. The precision of imatinib's action is astounding. It targets just one single molecule out of hundreds in the network enclosed within the bone marrow cells and suppresses it, which translates into the clinical symptoms subsiding and a remission of the illness.

These sensational results in treating myeloid leukemia have opened the gates wide for further experiments of this kind. Particular attention is being paid to other proliferative blood diseases, defined by the term "myeloproliferative syndromes." They are characterized by excessive production within the bone marrow of mature erythrocytes (*polycythemia vera*), thrombocytes (*thrombocythemia essentiale*) or collagen fibers (*myelofibrosis*). In 2005–2007 it was discovered that at the foundation of these long-recognized, classic diseases lies an acquired mutation of the gene that codes a certain element of the signals' paths. In technical terms, this element is the protein kinase JANUS 2, and thus it is a particle from a broadly understood family of transmitters, whose malfunction we encountered in myeloid leukemia. We have not yet identified a drug that might suppress it or regulate its connections with other paths (as implied by its "Janus" face). But once they become accessible, the treatment of blood cancers will really be transformed into selective, targeted therapy. Meanwhile, the search continues for mutations in other kinases. In 2007, five hundred and eighteen genes coding protein kinases in two hundred and ten cancer patients were examined, and about a thousand mutations were discovered. However, it is incredibly hard to judge their role in initiating cancer, because the genes that we research once the illness has already been diagnosed contain millions of cells with mutant DNA. Some of these mutations have arisen under the influence of the first malfunctions and play a role in the growth and spread of the tumor. They are like "drivers"; others are accidental mutations, and they are called "passengers." In some forms of lung cancer (the so-called non-small-cell form) permanent damage occurs on the surface of a particular receptor. Drugs are already in clinical trials that aim to curb a hyperactive receptor, defined for short as the EGFR (epidermal growth factor receptor). In some patients an improvement is successfully achieved, and in others, after some time, resistance develops and a new mutation emerges. These observations are still relatively rare and short-lived. This field of activity is the focus of interest for the pharmaceuticals industry, because the receptor is the beginning of the signals' paths.

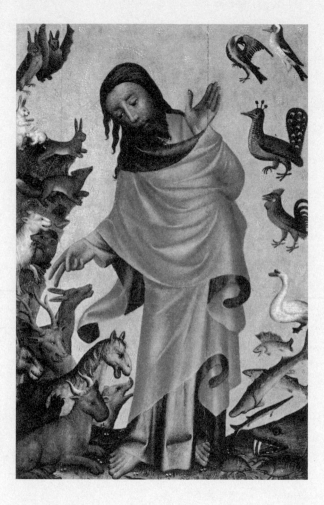

Master Bertram
Creation of the Animals, 1383
Kunsthalle, Hamburg

THE TRUTHS OF BIOLOGY AND FAITH

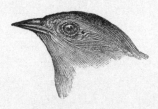

"There are two popular myths about Charles Darwin," wrote John Gribbin, "neither of which resembles the truth." The first is that Darwin was a young dilettante, an English gentleman who had the fortune to be taken on a journey around the world, during which he saw some fairly obvious evidence of evolution in action and suggested an explanation that any intellectual of his era could have thought of in those circumstances. The second myth tells of a rare genius, who in an exceptional flash of intuition pushed science forward whole generations. In reality, Charles Darwin and his ideas about natural selection "were very much products of their time, but he was unusually hard working, painstaking and persistent in his search for scientific truth across a wide range of disciplines."

At the age of twenty-two, after graduating from Cambridge, he embarked, as a naturalist, on the three-masted *HMS Beagle*, a ten-gun brig whose task was to map the coast of South America. He later defined this as "the most important event of my life." He spent five years on the voyage, and sailed right around the world. He had open eyes, a clever outlook and a curious mind. The South

American coast, all the way to Tierra del Fuego, which the ship remained alongside for weeks on end, revealed to him successive biological formations and rock layers—with fossils—piled on top of each other. They provided original illustrations for the recently published *Principles of Geology* by Charles Lyell, which Darwin took with him on the voyage and about which he later wrote with admirable frankness: "I always feel as if my books came half out of Lyell's brain, and that I have never acknowledged this sufficiently ..." In Chile he experienced an earthquake, which made him aware of the formational power of tectonic movements. He made close observations, and described the fauna and flora he encountered, including some unusual animals, such as ostrich-like birds. He visited the Galapagos Islands—an archipelago lying over one thousand kilometers from the South American continent that, in view of this distance, experienced selective colonization by only a few living organisms, which then underwent the process of evolution. And there, on the Galapagos, at the sailors' traditional feasts, he enjoyed dining on large turtles, accepting with good faith the general view that earlier travelers had congregated them there to provide food for their successors. Only once they had sailed onward did he start to wonder about certain differences between the turtles inhabiting neighboring, separate islands, and about the variability of the chaffinches that he noticed and described extremely precisely—in short, about varying features of related species. By the time he reached the shores of England, he was already strongly convinced of the existence of evolution.

But, of course, Darwin did not "invent" or discover evolution. The ancient Greeks considered it, and several decades before Darwin, Jean-Baptiste Lamarck presented the theory of evolution in detail and formulated its four laws, of which the most famous one, about the "inheritance of acquired characters" as the motor for changes, turned out to be untrue. Another evolutionist was

Lamarck's contemporary, Charles Darwin's grandfather Erasmus Darwin, who did not, apparently, know the great Frenchman's works. He was a lively character, seething with energy that found an outlet in all sorts of activities. A successful doctor with a flourishing practice, he fathered fourteen children born of two marriages (and not just), and was a friend to the brilliant scholars and poets of the era, founder of a debating club that with a sense of humor he christened the Lunar Society, patron for the construction of mills and canals, and a zealous opponent of slavery. He translated the whole of Linnaeus into English, and expressed his love of botany in verse, in a long work entitled *The Loves of the Plants*. In it he "literally made plants sexy," and charmed a wide audience. He also published scientific works that led to his being made a member of the Royal Society.

In *The Temple of Nature* he described evolution in verse—from microscopic specks to a wealth of life forms. He expressed the belief that the whole of life on Earth could come from one single, common ancestor. In extensive footnotes he gave numerous examples of the variability of species. He paid attention to the way features are shaped within the conditions of plant and animal husbandry, for example, how the speed and jumping ability of racehorses is increased, or the productivity of cereal crops is raised by skillful cross-breeding, and thus by (artificial) selection. In its developed form, this idea was the central concept within his grandson's theory.

Not long after returning to England, Charles Darwin bought a house and garden at Down in the county of Kent. We can see him there, as every day, for years on end, he walks along a gravel path in the garden, considering evolution. He compiles and records in his notebooks a wealth of evidence for its presence and authenticity. In his spare time he breeds and crosses pigeons, and writes insightful treatises on zoology, which guarantee him recognition among the experts and high status as a scientist. In autumn 1838 he picks up the sixth edition of a famous book by the British professor of political economy, Thomas Malthus. In it he reads that although the natural increase of people and mammals happens in geometrical progression, the number of adult individuals in the population remains at a stable level, because it is conditioned by limited access to food, death in the clutches of predators, wars and epidemics. And so Darwin finds the essential components of his theory about the mechanism of evolution—a struggle for survival among individuals of the same species, the result of which is that the best adapted survive. He sketched out these ideas immediately after reading Malthus, and wrote them down in detail in a private notebook dated 1842.

He acquainted only a small number of people with the results of his research and his reflections. He knew that the critics would devour him if he presented his life's work in a poorly documented way. This had been the fate of a book promoting evolution, published under a pseudonym by Robert Chambers. Above all Darwin felt that if he published his theory, it would upset the order of Victorian England, the stability of this world that had its foundations in the biblical Genesis—in short, it would go against the truths of religion. And so he described a letter to his friend the botanist Joseph Hooker, presenting the basic points of his theory of evolution and natural selection, as "like confessing a murder." Darwin waited twenty years, and the theory might only have seen the light of day after his death if not for a letter that reached him from the Antipodes in June 1858, and that came like a thunderbolt out of the blue. The author was named Alfred Russel Wallace. With the letter he enclosed a short manuscript. Darwin later said he could hardly have written a better abstract of his ideas himself.

There was one difference between them: property. Unlike Darwin, Wallace came from a poor family and from his early years had had to try to earn a living and help his siblings. They were united by the idea of evolution, the search for proof of it at the ends of the world, and some identical, though mutually independent explanations for its mechanism, derived from the same inspiration. Fifteen years younger than Darwin, Wallace was sure about evolution and set off to seek evidence of it in the jungles of Brazil. He spent four years there, collecting butterfly specimens in order to sell them at home, because exotic collecting had started to be fashionable after Darwin's publication of his description of his voyage on the Beagle. The ship he came home on sank. He lost his brother as well as the entire collection, and after ten days he was fished out of the sea. But soon after he set off for the Far East, having earlier very briefly met Darwin, with whom he maintained a sporadic correspondence. Laid low by a severe fever in the Moluccas, he remembered reading Malthus's book years earlier and had a revelation, saw the explanation for the mechanism of evolution and sent his letter to Darwin. The rest is history. Darwin's friends presented the letter at a session of the Linnaean Society in London along with Darwin's personal notebooks, written years earlier and guaranteeing him chronological precedence. Both studies were published together shortly after; Wallace had no objection to this solution. A year later Darwin published his life's work: *On the Origin of Species by Means of Natural Selection, or the Preservation of Favoured Races in the Struggle for Life*.

In his 2003 Harvey oration at the Royal College of Physicians, Sir Paul Nurse presented the four great ideas that form the core of biology and medicine. The first is the cell — the building material of life and the smallest brick to demonstrate its features by itself. Just like the other three great ideas, this one too took shape in the nineteenth century, and we owe its discovery to technical progress. In 1665 Robert Hooke pointed the eyepiece of the first microscope, which he had produced, at a sliver of cork. He saw some closed, adjoining, regular cavities to which he gave the Latin name *cella*, or cell. For a long time no one understood where the cells of plants and animals came from, until finally it was realized that they develop from the division of one, already existing cell into two descendants (*omnis cellula e cellula* — "every cell originates from another cell"). The cell is the atom of biology. We owe it respect, considering the fact that every one of us was once a single cell!

The second idea is genes — the elements of inheritance, carriers of information and components of the double helix of DNA, which is capable of self-duplication. The third is the idea that the vital processes can be understood as chemical reactions. Until the time of Louis Pasteur, there was much debate about the mysterious, unearthly and elusive life force (*vis vitalis*) — the source of our inner energy. When its enigmatic batteries weakened, life was extinguished. Pasteur's work on the fermentation of wine led him to conclude that chemical reactions are an expression of life. Thousands of chemical reactions controlled by biocatalysts, in other words, enzymes, are happening in each of our cells all the time. In them we find the explanation for the phenomena of life. In them the *vis vitalis* that had been sought for centuries materialized at last.

And finally the fourth idea is evolution. "Nothing in biology makes sense except in the light of evolution." It is the only thing that gives meaning to biology. Nonetheless, at first sight it looks as if evolution, being "essentially a historical theory," has lesser implications for clinical medicine than the other three ideas do, on which modern molecular medicine is based. But there is an exception: cancer. It develops when the genes controlling the growth and division of cells undergo damage or rearrangement. Unrestrained growth follows, and the proliferation of cells. This is an example of evolution by means of natural selection, happening at the cellular level within the human organism. Just as it happens in evolution at the level of the population, pre-cancerous or cancerous cells win the fight and supplant all others. The system has three features of evolution: reproduction, inheritance and genetic diversity. Isn't it a paradox that the same mechanisms that enabled the evolution of human life are also responsible for one of mankind's most dangerous diseases?

The opposite of fighting is symbiosis. We talk of it when two organisms coexist and closely cooperate, to their mutual advantage. In extreme cases they unite to form a single, new creature, and endosymbiosis takes place. Thus billions of years ago, at the beginning of evolution, the progenitor of today's cells (eukaryotes) took inside freely living bacteria, and they have survived to this day as separate structures. They are in every human and animal cell, where they are called mitochondria, and in every plant cell, where they are called chloroplasts. They have their own, circular DNA, different from the double helix of DNA enclosed in the nucleus, and they are ideally integrated with the cell, fulfilling important vital functions within it. As soon as endosymbiosis was accomplished, part of the newcomer's genes must have made its way into the host's DNA, into the cell's nucleus. We do not know if it was a mass influx, or a gradual permeation. We do know that this sort of transfer still occurs from time to time nowadays (though our information on this topic is extremely scant).

But the first nuclear cell was supposedly born by way of endosymbiosis too. Of course it was much earlier, before mitochondria and chloroplasts came into being. But when exactly? The scientists are still arguing about it. The time period under consideration is vast: from a little less than one billion to three-and-a-half billion years. Until recently they thought that in an extremely remote era lost in the mists of time, a prokaryote, or non-nuclear cell, turn itself into a eukaryote, or nuclear cell. These days, this concept is less well accepted. Let us suppose that at the very beginning of life, from one primogenitor two strains developed: eubacteria and archaebacteria. The latter were recognized as a separate group only a few years ago. They are single-celled organisms adapted to life in extreme environments (for example, extremely high temperatures). In 1975 Lynn Margulis put forward a now generally accepted hypothesis about "symbiogenesis" — the symbiotic origin of life. It says that the first nuclear cell came into being by way of symbiosis, through the combination of the above-mentioned primogenitors, built of cells without a nucleus.

The transfer of genes apparently played a crucial role in this process. It proved to be not at all accidental. In the nuclear cell, the so-called information genes (concerning the function of the nucleus) come from archaebacteria, while the so-called operational genes (controlling the function of the cytoplasm) come from eubacteria. This segregation, with the simultaneous elimination of whole large groups of genes, remains "one of the greatest enigmas in biology." And yet even today, after so many billions of years, the transfer of genes between species is common — among bacteria. Retroviruses and transposons act as go-betweens in transferring genes, in other words, in the direct migration of the DNA sequence from one species to another.

The genesis of the cell equipped with a nucleus, with developed substructures within the cytoplasm, remains "one of the most mysterious questions raised by eukaryotic genesis." Indeed, it concerns living organisms, eukaryotes characterized by a nucleus and counted among the five kingdoms: animals, plants, protozoa, fungi and myxophyta. In a radical development of Margulis's hypothesis, the diversification of species "is not due to random events and accepted neo-Darwinian processes, such as mutations and natural selection acting through competition and sexual selection on variants among members of one single species . . . Darwin was wrong . . . cooperation and symbiosis drive evolution." So the argument continues about the driving force of evolution.

Long before Darwin, Western thought shaped a great chain of existence, an organized, linear continuation. It took its beginning from inanimate rocks, moved on to plants, and from them to animals, and then man, and then turned towards the sky — and with the help of the angels — reached its limit in God. It was rich in details: it placed man above the monkeys and ascribed defined positions to the human races. It even foresaw, long before the discovery of the microscope, the world of invisible creatures, beings occupying the space between the animate and inanimate worlds. This image, this *scala naturae*, has been with us for centuries, and although the advocates of evolution have stripped it of its supernatural peak, it still remains with us. And it doesn't matter if we are moving from the lowest rungs upwards or in the opposite direction, as in the journey Richard Dawkins took us on in his book entitled *The Ancestor's Tale*. For the medieval theologian, this journey would have led to a tour of successive links in the well-known chain of existence, "albeit with some novelties and the startling omission of God."

The icon of evolution is the tree, which ironically has associations with the biblical Tree of Life. We draw it with very thin lines to fit in a large number of branches and twigs, on which we locate species and families of living things. In marking the spot and placing each life form, we are guided by similarity — nowadays, not so much external as genetic — because we believe that the history of evolution on Earth is contained within the genomes. We carry a chronicle of past events inside us. Even if it is a palimpsest — an ancient manuscript on parchment, where some of the older sentences have been scratched out or effaced — it is in this semantically multilayered text that hidden meanings shine through from behind the literal meaning. Reconstructing the history of living things is like recreating the history of languages. It brings the sort of amazement that Sir William Jones, a British lawyer in the Indies, must have felt, when in about 1780 he noticed the similarity between Sanskrit—which had not been a spoken language for centuries—and Latin and Greek. As he showed in his further research, these similarities extend to the Celtic languages, French, English, and . . . Polish. He realized that all the Indo-European languages, as he called them, are derived from a common source, which seemed to have appeared about seven to ten thousand years ago in Turkish Anatolia or on the steppes of southern Russia. "The resemblance between German and Dutch is comparable to that between any pair of mammals. Human and chimpanzee DNA are so similar, they are like English spoken in two slightly different accents." The roots of the English language have a Germanic origin. After 1066, however, English acquired many Romance words from Old French, made borrowings and thus underwent endosymbiosis! It is endosymbiosis and the horizontal transfer of genes that start to cause problems in reconstructing the tree of evolution. Horizontal rings start to implant themselves into the dominant vertical—of a tree, a ladder or a chain—and we start to hear voices saying that we should talk of the "ring of life" instead of the tree of life, or at least remember that the tree grew out of a ring.

We—the human beings, the leading pack—sit at the crown of the tree, at its very top. "We have a deep psychological need to see ourselves as the culmination of creation." For we could boldly present other versions of the branching tree of evolution without placing ourselves at the top, while still remaining in total agreement with modern genetic analyses. Our closest neighbor is the chimpanzee.

We must have shared a common ancestor five to seven million years ago, before he went his way, and we went ours.

Only 1.2 percent of human DNA is different from that of a chimp. Only? That is no small amount — exchanging one in a hundred bases within a nucleotide can affect thousands of genes, and this influence is multiplied if other, often concomitant circumstances, defined as deletions and insertions, are taken into account. And even if we document these, let's say, forty million differences in the sequences between man and the chimpanzee, what does it mean? DNA is not a treasure-house full of knowledge. In my view we are heading for a return to long-debated features such as culture, language and technology, in whose development not just nature, but also upbringing, plays a role. Although we live in the age of the genome, let us not forget that man is something "more than DNA."

Our family, *Homo sapiens*, originates from Africa. Somewhere between fifty to two hundred thousand years ago, we all developed from a small African population of only ten thousand. "Thus, from the genomic perspective, we are all Africans, either living in Africa or in quite recent exile outside Africa." Having reached the European and Asian continents, thirty thousand years ago we displaced the Neanderthals, who had lived there for several hundred thousand years. Our similarities, or maybe even kinships with them, will soon be estimable thanks to the elaboration of new genetic techniques. The first analyses of a million nucleotide bases from the remains of Neanderthal man was conducted in early 2007. From them it emerges that the DNA of man and Neanderthal man must have separated about half a million years ago. Curiously, like *Homo sapiens*, the Neanderthals apparently developed from a small group of only several thousand people.

❖❖❖

Evolution has become the fundamental law of biology, and we have a tendency to look at it as if it were a solid, unshakable construction, a mighty edifice. Of course, as science makes progress we do replace some of the blocks in this building, but we still see the same edifice. And yet thirty years ago a young British zoologist, Richard Dawkins, decided to change our point of view. In the introduction to his book *The Selfish Gene*, he wrote: "We are survival machines, robot vehicles blindly programmed to preserve the selfish molecules known as genes. This is a truth which still fills me with astonishment." Thanks to literary talent of a high order, clarity of thought and logical argumentation, he has broadcast his astonishment not only to scientists, but also to a wide audience of non-specialists.

It was recently said, though perhaps it is an exaggeration, that "*The Selfish Gene* has been, and remains, one of the most influential science books of all times." In this and subsequent books, Dawkins consolidated some new, not widely circulated ideas from the biology of the 1960s and 1970s, imbued them with his enthusiasm and dressed them in brilliant words. He presented evolution from the viewpoint of the gene, and drew conclusions from it. The image that appeared before our eyes is indeed remote from everyday, commonsense ontology. In a natural way we believe that the behavior and conduct of the individual are driven by impulse, self-interest, profit, love and maybe curiosity. We are inclined to transfer this interpretation to entire communities of people, to society as a whole. Meanwhile we were only meant to be reservoirs and carriers of genes that fight ruthlessly to survive, conquer their rivals and multiply in successive generations. This is the logic of Darwin, who to explain the order of Nature, its design — without a designer — proposed the concept of natural selection. Dawkins has extrapolated this concept at the submicroscopic level, where replicators, in other words genes, are formed.

But nowadays, thirty years since their publication and with the phenomenal development of molecular genetics, aren't Dawkins's ideas old hat? Not at all, since his central thought concerns how natural selection works, and not individual genes. Nevertheless, "many of the fundamental questions about evolution are almost as far from being answered now as they were in 1976."

These unsolved enigmas include altruism. Within the animal world human societies represent a huge anomaly, because they are characterized by the division of labor and cooperation between large groups of people who are not related by blood. States, or international global organizations, are a distinct example of this, but even primitive societies provide similar examples, such as communities with a dense network of barter relationships, communal hunting and fighting and sharing out food. It would be hard to find this sort of behavior among animals, even among the primates that are closely related to us. The exceptions include some insect societies (such as bees, or ants) and one species of mole. The altruistic behavior of worker bees, which have lost the capacity to reproduce and dedicate their lives to the community of the hive, kept Darwin awake at night. In it he saw "a special difficulty, which at first appeared to me insuperable, and actually fatal to the whole theory." Later he explained it as "family selection," and even nowadays it is thought to be based on genetic kinship. Research into altruism related to kinship has had a rich development, producing sociobiology and even leading to attempts to encapsulate the enigma within a mathematical equation, called Hamilton's equation ($rB > C$, where r is the coefficient of kinship, B is profit, and C is cost).

However, human altruism seems to be distinct. The disinterested desire to share with others is the essence of humanity. It provides food for thought for philosophers, ethicists, biologists and even economists. The latter define altruism as "costly acts that confer economic benefits on other individuals." Diagnostic imaging of the brain indicates that the capacity to help others without expecting a reward can be inscribed permanently in our minds. We are starting to talk of the charity center and even trying to define its exact position in the "posterior superior temporal cortex." The more it is stimulated, the greater the chances that we will do something disinterestedly. In Mother Teresa of Calcutta, this spot in the brain must have shone brightly, dazzlingly, without the help of magnetic resonance imaging. And so medicine tells us that good deeds are born in the head (not forgetting the heart), but not in the genes. "Current gene-based evolutionary theories cannot explain important patterns of human altruism."

So does evolution justify our egoism and selfishness? Indeed it does, seen from the point of view of the "selfish genes." This very powerful metaphor has stamped itself on modern evolutionism, further deepening the resistance put up against it in some environments. Today, "fifty-four percent of U.S. adults believe that humans did not develop from an earlier species." This percentage is rising at an alarming rate, as in 1994 it was only forty-six. And so evolution, the greatest theory in biology, is engendering the greatest resistance since it was first fully portrayed in Darwin's work. Why is this happening? It is hard to find a more expressive answer than the reaction of Darwin's beloved wife, Emma. When he revealed his theory of evolution to her in secret not long before publishing it, she was not shocked by the boldness of the idea or the trouble it was likely to cause. But upon hearing the theory she burst into tears and became depressed, because it made her realize that after death she and her husband would no longer be together, for there would be no other world and everything would finish with death.

The theory of evolution deprived us of our unique status. It traced the long chain of our ancestors from animals, and pointed out our close connections with anthropoid apes. It is hard to come to terms with this idea, even for a child. When my younger son Wojtek was six, in an effort to introduce him to the mysteries of evolution, a student friend of ours said: "You know, Wojtek, monkeys are our relatives." "*Your* relatives?" asked the little boy in amazement. He knew his own relatives, and they didn't include any monkeys!

Wojtek did not grow up to be a creationist, and I don't think the creationists have missed him — there are quite enough of them. And if so, may we ask what it is that they and others find so offensive about the theory of evolution? The author of these words, though he is far from creationism, offends them with the metaphors he uses. Struggle, egoism, success, profit and loss, selfishness, ruthlessness, the triumph of the fittest — these words come up again and again in articles and books by the leading modern biologists. But of course that is just a matter of taste, with no real bearing on our perception of the theory. We find the proper answer in the claim that no one and nothing have made such a large contribution to the secularization of western societies as Darwin and his theory of evolution. "Darwin made it possible to be an intellectually fulfilled atheist," wrote Dawkins. And in subsequent years he added: "I'm a Darwinist, because I believe the only alternatives are Lamarckism or God, neither of which does the job as an explanatory principle." As science stands on the footing of Darwinism, its implications are profound and wide-ranging: "The universe we observe has precisely the properties we should expect if there is, at bottom, no design, no purpose, no evil and no good, nothing but blind pitiless indifference." In the part relating to the values of good and evil, these words lead us to the Book of Genesis. And we might well ask for a joke, don't they attest, in the work of an eminent geneticist, to the inheritance of original sin? Once he had plucked the forbidden fruit in Paradise, man began to decide for himself, without God's help, what was good and what was evil. The sin of the first parents' disobedience passes from generation to generation, just as if each generation had repeated that gesture of picking the apple — original sin, an inherited feature that does not mutate. Where, in what gene can we find it in Dawkins, but also in every one of us?

However, the world as presented by the geneticists gives us nothing to laugh about. What an alien, hostile place it is! As Czesław Miłosz asks:

> Have we really lost faith in that other space?
> Have they vanished forever, both Heaven and Hell?

A jumble of battling genes is a diabolical vision. Indeed, "the devil," a word ultimately derived from the Greek *dia-bolos*, means the one who separates, disunites. Evil lies in dispersion and fragmentation, which opposes our longing for integrity. It is that alienation that isolates man from man and man from God. Hellfire burned for centuries in grates and furnaces, and now hell seems to have taken root inside us, "in our serfdom, in our defenselessness in the face of the natural forces residing within us — nowadays the domains of the biologist, doctor and psychiatrist." It is doubtful whether the doctor, even by turning to squirming genes, would have the power to extinguish the flames consuming us.

What a pity, wrote one reviewer of Richard Dawkins's book, *The God Delusion*, that in his radical argument with the evidence for the existence of God, the author is "so easily in opposition to the quest for spiritual meaning in life." Because while evolution can tell us a lot about how life developed, it cannot answer the profound question about the meaning of life, or why the universe exists. The opinions so heatedly expressed by the British "Darwinian fundamentalist," also known as "Darwin's Rottweiler," have stirred some opposition. The American scientist Francis Collins, head of the team that performed the gigantic task of decoding the entire human genome, letter by letter, has joined the debate. The result of his work, the recording itself, is a weighty piece of evidence for the authenticity of the theory of evolution. Yes, replies Collins, but it was God who used the mechanism of evolution to create human beings. So he advocates evolutionary theology, in which God does not unambiguously determine the far-flung conditions of the universe, but "makes man His confidant, responsible for the future form of the work of creation." Dawkins ridicules Collins for being "anti-scientific," while others see in his attitude a desire to cast bridges across the chasm dividing intellectuals from ordinary Americans, for whom religion, we are tempted to say, is written in their genes.

And so some find proof of God's non-existence in the theory of evolution, while others find quite the opposite, a sign of His presence. But is that really the right place to look for Him? Within the reasoning of — albeit brilliant — geneticists and biologists? Is it the task of reason to issue opinions on the meaning of faith? There are two orders of knowledge: one that is appropriate to reason and one that is appropriate to faith. For the truth that we approach by an empirical route, by perceiving it with the senses, reason is the light. Alongside it exists the truth that passes beyond the limits of experience, in search of the meaning of existence, opening the way to the metaphysical dimension of reality, summoning us to the absolute and to transcendence—the truth of faith. What is the relationship between them? As Tertullian asked: "What does Athens have in common with Jerusalem? The Academy with the Church?"

There have been various replies to this question. Until the late Middle Ages, there was thought to be a bond between them. Thomas Aquinas wrote of the harmony between reason and faith, about their profound unity. In the centuries that followed, this unity was shaken until it broke—thanks to systems that declared themselves on the side of rational cognition, divorced from faith and offering the only alternative to it. In such cases the theory of evolution was often put forward as an example. However, biological evolution cannot be the touchstone for the existence or nonexistence of God. It is logically inscribed into the image of the world as drawn by modern cosmology, which is a thoroughly evolutionary image, starting from the Big Bang. Also clear is the attitude of the Holy See, as expressed in a famous letter from John Paul II to the Papal Academy of Sciences and summed up in the sentence: "The scientific theory of evolution is not at odds with any truth of the Christian faith."

The two orders of knowledge do not have to be at odds with each other. They are joined by a deep bond, and they lead to the unity of truth, to its completeness. Reason casts light on the world in which we live, and faith gives it meaning. Because "meaning," wrote Leszek Kołakowski, "comes only from the *sacrum*, because no empirical research can produce it." John Paul II expressed this deep bond in these beautiful words: "Faith and reason (*fides et ratio*) are like two wings on which the human spirit rises to the contemplation of the truth."

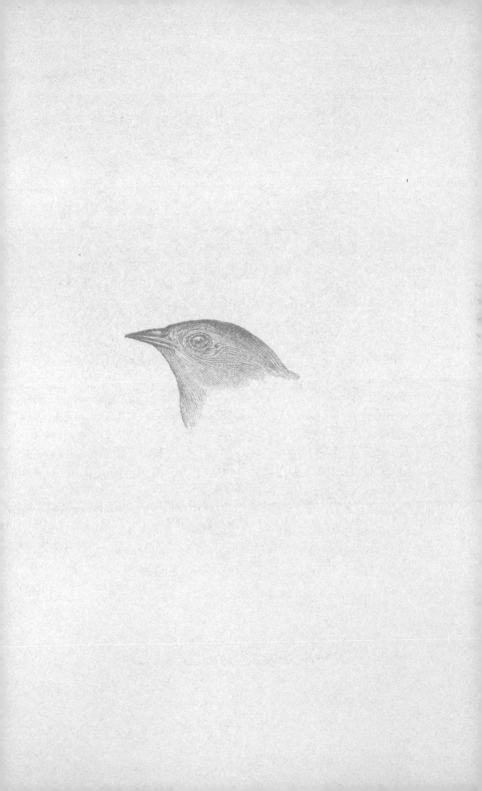

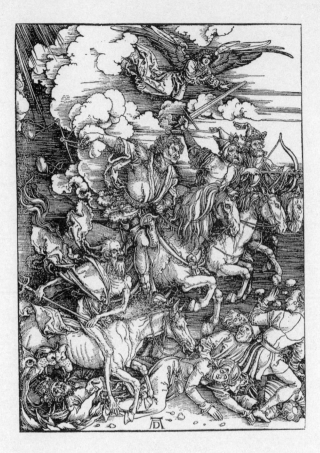

Albrecht Dürer
Four Horsemen of the Apocalypse, 1498
woodcut

THE BORDERLANDS

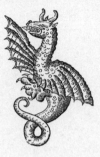

The picture in my school biology textbook showed a small, flat, rectangular box, with a broad, checked pattern on its surface. Now that I think about it, this pattern could only have been various shades of gray superimposed on the poor-quality, fuzzy reproduction of the picture that recorded itself in my memory with such crystal clarity, so sharply. This crystal, the little box with the perfect cuboid shapes, was the tobacco mosaic virus. The caption under the picture left no doubt about it. However, from that moment I started having doubts. How could a crystal like that one go on and on lasting for months, or even years, and then one day "come to life" on some tobacco leaves? And while it was lasting in that way, wasn't it alive? Could it have sunk into deep hibernation, as some animals do in winter? Did it pass from inanimate to animate form when it started to replicate on the leaves, like a tiny parasite? "In principle," said our biology teacher, "viruses are not alive." But that did not dispel my doubts, even though in those years we were taught at school that life can arise from inanimate material. Hadn't Olga Lepeshinskaya, the Soviet scientist, obtained cells in a test tube by mixing and heating simple chemical compounds, and hadn't Joseph Vissarionovich Stalin himself confirmed the accuracy of her experiments at a plenum of the Central Committee of the Communist Party of the Soviet Union? The border of life had lost its focus if a (Soviet) person was able to create cells resulting from the simplest, dead building bricks.

The memory of my youthful quandaries was unexpectedly brought back to life in 2005 because of a letter by one of the American molecular biologists to the journal *Nature*. He writes that after sequencing hundreds of flu viruses, he keeps realizing that he and his colleagues talk about viruses as living organisms. And yet in scientific publications they are careful to write "particle" and not "cell," and "segment" but not "chromosome." These latter definitions are indeed reserved for living organisms, and although he went to school in the other hemisphere twenty or thirty years after me, the author was also taught that viruses are not alive. It is easier to swallow that in the case of the tiny flu virus, which is equipped with barely eleven genes, but what are we to do with the recently discovered giant called the "mimivirus," which inhabits (not to say "lives in") amoebas? It has a double helix of DNA —just as we do (though a shorter one, of course) complex mechanisms that serve to repair it and dozens of genes never encountered in viruses before. Amazed by the wealth of its structure, the discoverers of the mimivirus put forward the intriguing hypothesis that viruses are one of the earliest offshoots of the genealogical tree of life. With the passage of time they have lost many of their genes and come to rely entirely on their hosts. If this is true, how many genes have to be lost for an organism to stop being called live?

The question about the definition of life appears in a new light because of the reconstruction of the Spanish flu virus. It was the

cause of the most terrible pandemic in history, which erupted in
1918 and claimed about a hundred million victims. The first news of
the deadly wave of flu was blocked by the British, French and German military censors. Reports about it could only appear in Spain,
a neutral country. As only the Spanish press was writing about the
epidemic, it was called "Spanish flu." In its first twenty-five weeks
it killed more people than AIDS did in twenty-five years, and in
one year it killed more than the Black Death (or plague) in an entire
century. After a year it began to subside, and after two it died out,
perhaps because the microbe, which remained unidentified for a
long time after, had mutated and lost its virulence. Over eighty
years later a detailed analysis of the virus was performed, the virus
having been obtained from the remains of three people claimed by
the Spanish flu. These included an Inuit woman lying in the eternal
ice of Alaska. Small pieces of the virus that killed her were extracted
from the remains of her lungs, and from them its entire DNA was
reconstructed. Then it was introduced into some human kidney
cells cultivated in vitro, where it converted itself into hundreds of
descendant particles. Their virulence went way beyond imagination. When the virus was injected into mice, after four days their
lungs contained thirty-nine thousand times more Spanish flu particles than after infection with an ordinary flu virus. Six days after
being infected, not a single mouse was still alive.

Isn't the word "resurrection" appropriate here? "Risen from the
dead"? The virus was dead. Its remains were still there in the preserved lungs of the Inuit woman, scattered, disintegrated fragments
of genetic material, RNA. Using the classic methods of molecular biology, they were changed into DNA, their composition was
established and the tiny pieces obtained were joined together into a
full genome sequence, which served as a model for laboratory synthesis of the viral DNA. Two years earlier, on the basis of similar
principles, in another laboratory scientists created artificial phage, a

virus that attacks bacteria. Small synthetic fragments of DNA were "sewn" together into the phage genome, built up of five thousand, four hundred pairs of bases. It attacked bacteria and behaved in every respect just like its naturally produced namesake.

Thus the Spanish flu virus "arose from the dead," but was it now alive? In any case, it killed. How dangerous it can be was a known fact when the scientists set about "resurrecting" it. The laboratory where it was done was one of the best-guarded places in the United States. Apart from all the essential cautionary measures and guarantees against the virus "escaping," only three people had access to it, and their fingerprints and retinal images were checked each time, once they had passed through a series of protective chambers. The pessimists conjure up dark visions of the Spanish flu virus sooner or later getting into the hands of bio-terrorists, who if necessary might even be tempted to recreate it themselves, since its DNA has been published. The optimists stress that precise knowledge of the construction of the Spanish flu virus, and being able to define the mutation that distinguishes it from all other flu viruses, will not only help us to track the future threats we are always hearing about, but will also provide the basis for developing effective vaccines.

The markets of Southeast Asia are a breeding ground for flu microbes, with their crowded stalls selling edible birds, pigs, dogs and other animals, both domestic as well as semi-feral. It is there that a mutant of avian flu was able to develop, capable of penetrating the human organism very easily, and so did the chimera virus that combines the genes of the microbes that cause avian and human flu. News from there of sporadic flare-ups of infection are received with close attention and fear—the same fear that remains somewhere deep inside us from the days of the Spanish flu, and no doubt even earlier, from more than six centuries ago, when the Black Death sailed into Europe on ships also from East Asia.

+ + +

When a new pandemic suddenly struck in the early 1980s, it came from a completely different direction. In 1981 a rare type of pneumonia and other unusual infections were described in five young homosexuals. In the months that followed, the reports began to multiply. Drug addicts who used syringes, hemophiliacs and other people receiving blood transfusions — including women and children too — were falling victim to the disease, which invariably ended in death. Many possible causes were considered, including mycosis infections and poisoning by chemical substances. In the years 1983 to 1984 the virus was discovered, and it was established that it caused AIDS. The path to this success bristled with special difficulties, because in view of the infection's long incubation period, when the patients were examined, they "usually had numerous other infections." The original observations came from the Pasteur Institute, and their full development took place at the National Institutes of Health in the United States. For years a fierce public argument raged about precedence, until finally the two men who discovered the virus, Luc Montagnier of Paris and Roberto Gallo of Washington, shook hands. But before that the world had become paralyzed by fear. On television screens, movie stars, viewers' favorites, the rich and the famous kept appearing to bid this world farewell. They all left it amid suffering and a universal sense of helplessness, and their funerals turned into demonstrations against the injustice and cruelty of fate. For the first time in history, before spreading right around the world, a pandemic was already global, thanks to the media who reported on it every day in the news headlines. Only in the late 1980s were laboratory diagnostic tests devised and the first drugs introduced, which were initially not very effective. It was already known that the infection spreads mainly by means of sexual contact, and also through blood transfusions. In Poland, living behind sealed borders, in the gloomy shadow of martial law, we heard in disbelief the catastrophic news about the mysterious epidemic, and read about the hospital isolation wards that were popping up like mushrooms after rain, but where it had not been possible to help patients with AIDS in a radical way.

This virus is a cruel killer. It attacks the immune system and paralyzes resistance. Hence its name, HIV, for "Human Immunodeficiency Virus." The system of a patient with damaged immunity easily yields to opportunistic infections, in other words, the kind the immune system of a healthy person has no trouble coping with. The more was known about the virus, the more surprising it was, above all for its capacity to metamorphose. Because it kept changing, varying and mutating, again and again, in the course of a few hours even. It also rearranged its genes whenever it infected, as well as whenever it replicated itself. To replicate, it used the genetic mechanism of the cell it was attacking, because it carried enzymes enabling it to make itself a permanent part of its host's DNA. As the cells of the immune memory, in which the virus takes up residence, are situated within tissue reservoirs that are hard for drugs to access, it is virtually guaranteed immortality and a permanent supply of descendant viruses.

In 2005 an editorial appeared in *The Lancet* with the characteristic title: "Antiretroviral Therapy for HIV: Medical Miracles Do Happen." The title says it all. Indeed, a quarter of a century since the outbreak of the AIDS epidemic, we now have some highly effective drugs at our disposal, professionally known as antiretrovirals. They block the replication of HIV or stop it from fusing with cells. They minimize the danger of opportunistic illnesses, slow down the progress of the disease, reduce the risk of death and significantly prolong life. Simultaneous application of several of these drugs causes the virus to disappear from the blood and become undetectable by even the most sensitive methods, and the patient's immune system undergoes a notable degree of reconstruction. Although the treatment does not lead to a complete cure, because we are unable to eradicate the virus once it has integrated with the host's genome (its DNA), the patient's fate has completely changed, and the number of hospitalizations in centers specializing in treating AIDS is constantly decreasing. Highly sensitive diagnostic tests enable very early recognition of the illness, and the treatment protects against its progress and dangerous consequences.

So have we got the better of the AIDS epidemic? Not in the least. We only have to look at the figures. In the twenty-five years since the first five sufferers were described, about forty million people worldwide have become infected with the HIV virus. In the United States there are a million of them, of whom one in five or six do not know they are infected. Contact with these people is the conclusive cause of about forty thousand new infections each year. However, the hotbed of the infection is elsewhere. About two-thirds of the forty million people infected live in the countries of central and southern Africa. "Only one fifth of people in developing countries who need treatment are receiving antiretroviral therapy," whereas routine testing of blood donors that is of fundamental importance in overcoming the epidemic is still rarely performed there. Tuberculosis develops easily in AIDS sufferers, and in some African countries it already bears the hallmarks of an epidemic. There are justified fears that AIDS is violently gathering strength in Russia and India. Some say the tide of the epidemic is moving with a domino effect, where as one brick falls it topples the next few ahead of it. These bricks are countries that are developing, or to put it directly, poor. Meanwhile, medicine has brought hope to people living in the wealthy countries.

❖❖❖

In my student years, a visit from the Jehovah's Witnesses was not a rare event. There would be a ring at the door, and the neatly dressed person on the doorstep would start talking. Here they were with their good news, wanting to tell it, present it in all its splendor and gain a bridgehead, but we would immediately say we were not interested, so they would leave a thin brochure and an address with an invitation to a meeting, and the door was closed. In how many homes must it have been slammed in their faces the moment they started speaking? Who would want to listen to sectarians? But, never discouraged, next day off they went on their missionary outings again. We knew their faith forbade them to accept blood transfusions. This subject used to come up sporadically in hospital conversations when I was working as a young doctor. My boss reckoned we should respect the patient's wishes, and only do a transfusion if the patient lost consciousness, which from the ethical point of view, or simply in terms of logic, seemed to me dubious. Of course, we regarded the ban on transfusions as ignorant superstition, absurd nonsense. Doesn't blood save lives? But as I think about it years later, I can see that we might have found a good deal of common sense in the Jehovah's Witnesses' injunction, though in those days it was impossible to rationalize.

In the mid-twentieth century scientists began to realize that blood transfusions could cause hepatitis, colloquially known as infectious jaundice. The more transfusions, the greater the risk. And so in 1959 it was demonstrated in the United States that hepatitis developed in seventeen to one hundred percent of patients receiving transfusions. So doctors were obliged to be economical in their use of blood. But the demand was becoming enormous. In the 1960s and early 1970s came the rapid development of cardiac surgery, transplant surgery and kidney dialysis. Heart operations consumed liters of blood. And for the anesthesiologist, whenever the blood pressure fell dangerously towards the end of a long operation, or for the nephrologist, whenever the hemoglobin of a weakening, chronically dialyzed patient reached a third of its proper value, there was nothing simpler or more appropriate than to put the patients on a drip to feed blood into their veins. "The benefits were instantaneous; the harm invisible."

The cause of the hepatitis remained elusive. In 1965 Baruch Blumberg described a protein in the blood of a hemophiliac that reacted with the blood of an Australian Aborigine. The conjecture was put forward that the hemophiliac, treated many times with transfusions, was producing antibodies against something that had been present in the blood of one of his donors, and also in the blood of the Aborigine, with which he had never come into contact. This "something" was initially called the Australia antigen, and about a dozen years later it turned out to be the hepatitis B virus (*hepatitis viralis B*). So Australian Aborigines carry in their blood cells a "marker" (an antigen) that is deceptively similar to the "marker" for the virus, which is the cause of the blood reaction. Although using the blood of an Aborigine for the research was pure coincidence, Blumberg followed this lead, developed his observations and devised a test for detecting the Australia antigen, which in 1976 won him the Nobel Prize. The discovery was enthusiastically received, and the test was immediately introduced at blood donor centers. It looked as if hepatitis, as transferred by way of blood (from donors who carried the virus without being aware of their infection), had been brought under control. Yet a few years later it was confirmed that, when tested for the presence of the hepatitis B virus, thousands of patients receiving blood transfusions had developed it. Either the test was not sensitive enough, or there were yet other, unknown causes of hepatitis present in transfused blood. The medics began to talk rather awkwardly of "non-A, non-B" hepatitis, and the issue was eclipsed by the outbreak of the AIDS epidemic, whose virus was also transferred via blood. Only at the dawn of the 1990s were further hepatitis viruses discovered and cloned from blood, to be given the names of successive letters of the alphabet: C, D, E . . . Hepatitis C is a dangerous, chronic and common illness. It is estimated that in Poland the number of people infected is close to a million. Highly sensitive tests detecting carriers of these viruses are now obligatory at blood donor centers, and the number of infections is noticeably falling.

So blood transfusions have become safe. But are they entirely safe? Might they not hide yet other viruses, fortunately rare now? We cannot be sure. Maybe we should ask the Jehovah's Witnesses what they think? But they stopped knocking at my door a good many years ago.

Viruses have been with us since the dawn of history. The face of Ramses V, who died in 1157 BC, is covered in smallpox scars. Smallpox could also be counted as one of the great epidemics that plagued the ancient and medieval world right up to the eighteenth century, when Edward Jenner discovered a vaccine against it. As Aristotle wrote about rabies: "Dogs suffer from the madness. This causes them to become very irritable, and all animals they bite become diseased." And what about the dreadful polio virus, which paralyzes the nervous system? I remember some children from my first year as a medical student who were suffering from poliomyelitis. They lay without moving, shut in solid metal boxes, with only their heads sticking out at one end and their feet at the other. These "iron lungs" replaced their paralyzed respiratory muscles: they compressed air, and by pressing it against the rib cage, caused it to move regularly. Respirators had not yet been invented, and mass inoculations were introduced a few years later.

Many common illnesses prompted by viruses accompany us through life: measles, herpes, shingles, flu . . . So it is fair to suppose that viruses are the cause of other illnesses too, whose origin we do not know. I am thinking of one in particular: aspirin-induced asthma. It has as long a history as aspirin. In the first years after aspirin was introduced into health care, that is, in the early twentieth century, it was soon apparent that in some people it caused violent, dangerous asthma attacks. The breathlessness erupted so suddenly that quite often there was no time to get the patient to a hospital. It was not much easier for us to save such patients from their dyspnea seventy years later, at the start of my medical practice. The general belief was that it was an allergy to aspirin, but there was no proof. In the patients I treated, an asthma attack could be caused by not just aspirin, but by other painkillers too, such as pyralgin, indomethacin, or the then-popular fenoprofen. Their chemical structures were completely different, which put a question mark over their "sensitizing" effect on the road to allergy. At the time Ryszard Gryglewski and I developed an assumption that asthma attacks induced by aspirin had nothing to do with allergy, in other words the combination of the drug and a special antibody, but were caused by aspirin blocking—in the patients' lungs—a single enzyme called cyclooxygenase (COX). In making this hypothesis, we were inspired by the research of our friend and mentor, Sir John Vane, who later won the Nobel Prize. How do you try to prove such a hypothesis? We gathered a group of a few dozen patients who had experienced reactions to aspirin, and, with the help of Doctor Grażyna Czerniawska-Mysik, we gave them twenty-five different drugs, in increasing doses, starting from tiny bits of tablets, while keeping them under close observation and measuring the response of their bronchial tubes with the help of spirometry. We were afraid for our patients and sat with them for hours, while also knowing that proving our hypothesis would make it possible to prevent dangerous asthma attacks. Some drugs prompted reactions, but others did not; fortunately it all happened without any serious consequences. In the meantime, Gryglewski assessed whether the drugs we had tested have an effect in vitro on an incriminated enzyme. When we compared the results, to our joy it turned out that only drugs that blocked COX prompted a constriction of the bronchial tubes in the patients. Moreover, the intensity of the constriction was proportional to the strength of the effect of the drug in vitro. These results, which were then confirmed in many laboratories, led to the formation of the "theory of cyclooxygenase aspirin-induced asthma." It allows us to tell the patient precisely which drugs he categorically must not take, and which ones he can safely use in case of pain, fever or inflammation. Moreover, in the case of new drugs, the theory allows us to predict whether they are safe for aspirin-induced asthma patients or not.

So where are the viruses? In the patients in question, the dangerous reactions to aspirin and related drugs had developed in the course of their lives; there had been a time when they could take them without the slightest problem. The picture resulting from our analysis emerged just the same, regardless of whether it was happening in Poland, ten other European countries, Australia, Japan, Korea or Argentina. First a cold, then catarrh for months on end that refused to respond to treatment and finally persistent asthma, the attacks of which intensified after aspirin, but which progressed as usual even if the patient avoided aspirin. So aspirin was just the marker indicating the illness — one that is not at all rare (about ten percent of adult asthmatics suffer from it) and has an extremely characteristic course. What could have been causing it? We seek the sources of an illness at its beginnings. And it always starts the same way: with symptoms resembling flu. This prompted me to conjecture that the first cause of the illness might be a virus taking up permanent residence in the respiratory tract and causing a long-standing hidden infection. I suspected that it was one of the extensive family of rhinoviruses responsible for "colds." I looked for it in various ways but could not find it, until a colleague from our hospital, Professor Marek Sanak, devised a sensitive molecular technique enabling us to detect rhinoviruses in the bronchial tubes. We used it in experiments conducted jointly with Professor William Busse from the University of Wisconsin, Madison, and we concluded that there was a rhinovirus hidden in the wall of the bronchi in one hundred percent of all patients suffering from aspirin-induced asthma. But ... we were also finding it quite frequently in other types of asthma, and sometimes even in healthy people. It was the source of a hidden, enduring infection, as none of the people whom we tested had experienced a severe viral illness for at least a month before. But for the illness to be triggered and the cyclo-oxygenase function to be disturbed, did the virus need special environmental features or local disturbances in resistance that it could not find elsewhere? And was it actually this very virus? We do not know. I had come across a similar question earlier from my London colleagues who, after examining the specimens I had brought from the patients under an electron microscope, said: "All right, but what virus is it meant to be?" I did not know how to answer that question. But if we are familiar with what we are looking for, can we find something unfamiliar? Which does not change the fact that my search for the aspirin-induced asthma virus reminds me—at difficult moments—of the hunting of the Snark ... A creature of the imagination so distinctive that it starts to live its own life.

Viruses have turned out to be the cause of various infectious diseases, and have also revealed the mystery of cancer. It all began in 1909, when a hen breeder from Long Island called at the Rockefeller Institute in New York. His champion, a hen that had been showered in medals at various competitions, was sick. There was a tumor growing rapidly on her right breast. The breeder was looking for help, but the only man to take an interest in his troubles was a young researcher named Peyton Rous. How Rous persuaded the breeder to sacrifice the bird has remained his secret forever. He killed the hen and conducted two key experiments. Firstly, he transplanted cells from the tumor into a healthy chick. Secondly, he made an extract from the tumor, passed it through filters that retain bacteria and injected the resulting filtration into some healthy chicks, causing in them a tumor identical to the original one. Rous realized that he had discovered the virus that causes cancer (or to put it more precisely, sarcoma). However, at the time no one knew what a virus was. It was regarded as a poison (hence the Latin name *virus*) that seemed to live a life of its own. Then Rous changed the direction of his research, and this work was taken up by others. Among them I should mention the Polish scholar Ludwik Gross. Having got out of Poland in 1940, he conducted his research alone, in the difficult conditions of a Brooklyn hospital, and discovered the virus that causes leukemia in mice. But hopes of discovering the viruses causing leukemia in humans have proved futile. Nowadays we know of just one, rare form of human leukemia caused by a viral infection. But the wheels have been set in motion. And in the eighty-sixth year of his life Peyton Rous won the Nobel Prize.

In the early 1970s scientists confirmed that the virus discovered by Rous has four genes. It uses three of them for reproduction, but the fourth (called SRC) only initiates and maintains growth. It is this gene, they reckoned, that changes the course of a cell's life, switching it from normal growth to unrestrained cancerous proliferation. Rous's virus belongs to the retroviruses, in other words, it inscribes itself in the host's genome, integrating with it. So could the SRC gene be found in the genome of hens? The answer was positive. And in other birds, even those least related to hens, such as the emu or the ostrich? The answer was positive. And in other animals? Yes again. And in the human genome? There too. J. Michael Bishop and Harold Varmus, the two Nobel Prize winners to whom we owe the answers to these questions, have demonstrated that in our DNA we carry both SRC and many other genes known as proto-oncogenes. They lie dormant in our double helix and wake up when they undergo mutation or during the abnormal translocation of chromosomes or, finally, when the mechanisms that block their activity weaken. This awakening of the oncogenes is a feature of almost all cancers that attack man. And so a single cell divides into two descendants, these divide into the next ones and so on ad infinitum. The reference to infinity is apt. Some human cancers have been subjected in laboratories to so many passages in vitro for so many generations that "the number of cells produced exceeds the number of stars in the known universe."

And what about viruses? What is their connection with these phenomena? Nowadays, we reckon they progressed like pirates. They kidnapped from animal genomes (including the human genome for sure) proto-oncogenes, which were not of any special value to them. This piratical practice has revealed the mysteries of cancer to us. Dozens of years would have had to go by before we found these genes that actually initiate the development of cancers, buried deep in our genomes. Instead of that, we were handed them on a plate, as it were, displayed within the retroviruses, which had extracted them from the depths of our genomes and made them available for cancer research.

Viruses are linked with the genome, with DNA, by a mysterious bond. When a virus forces its way into a cell, it comes up against the DNA, which is far larger than itself, and is surprised to find some similarities. Some of its segments see themselves in the host's DNA as if in a mirror—they are its reflection. In places the similarities are so great that they make us think of a blood relationship. So, apart from the exchange of a few segments, like, for example, the proto-oncogenes described above, might they be linked by something else too? Yes, some suggest that "it was the virus that invented DNA." To imagine this, let us cast our minds back more than four billion years, to the time when life is supposed to have come into being on our planet. We are entering "the RNA world," in other words, a world where RNA already existed, but there was no DNA yet. These two basic carriers of genetic information have some significant differences. RNA — the single thread that in certain circumstances is able to catalyze chemical reactions, and even its own replication — is a more versatile but also a more fragile structure than the rigid DNA. In the primordial world, it was the dynamic RNA that took care of almost everything. It accelerated reactions and replications, which is now done by proteins, and gathered information, which is now gathered by DNA. It is hard to imagine the stiff structure made by the double helix of DNA multiplying itself with the help of a protein and being able to carry out all these numerous tasks. This is one of the reasons why it is supposed that DNA came later, after proteins had already enriched the world.

And here is a scenario with a virus in the main role. The virus, with its own DNA already formed, penetrates a primitive cell equipped only with RNA. With the help of an enzyme that it brings with it, so-called transcriptase, it makes copies of the DNA out of the cellular RNA. By doing this, it evades the cell's defenses and guarantees itself favorable conditions for survival. With the passage of time, using the mechanism offered by the virus, more and more genes shift from RNA to DNA. The cell perceives the benefit of the new, safe way of gathering information, and DNA becomes a constituent part of it.

However, there are scientists who do not cast a virus in the main role. They claim that DNA appeared before cell membranes had come into existence. And although all cells use it as a carrier of genetic information, they copy it in a different way, which has given rise to conjecture that DNA may have been "discovered" in the evolutionary process not just once, but many times. The origin of DNA stirs the imagination of scientists and is inciting increasingly lively debate. The enigmatic world of viruses is starting to occupy a prominent place in their minds. The diversity of viruses, their mobility, capacity for lightning-quick metamorphosis, agility and inventiveness in avoiding the defenses of the cell they are attacking astound and puzzle scientists. When we try to penetrate the dark corners of prehistory in our minds, to reach back to the time when life was being born, viruses look to us like invaders who came to conquer that world. They inoculated the conquered cells with their own culture, leaving them with DNA forever.

So what was there before the RNA world? When not even viruses existed yet? How did life emerge? Some seek its beginnings in excavations of the oldest rocks. Others conduct ingenious experiments in the conditions that must have reigned on Earth when life came into being. They dream of creating from scratch "a living chemical system" that faithfully imitates life ... and that is life. And here we start to tread on the shifting sands of the definition of life. For those who devote themselves to studying cell membranes, recreating those membranes in vitro is almost tantamount to solving the riddle of life. Other eminent experts on metabolism are convinced that the birth of life is connected with the emergence of the first metabolic cycle. And specialists in nucleic acids seek the origin in simpler structures than RNA, while information technology experts seek it in networks of artificial intelligence ... In August 2000 at a conference in Modena, scientists, philosophers and theologians discussed a single subject: "What is life?" On hearing the statements of the brilliant scholars, a leading American astrobiologist remembered the story about the elephant and the blind men. When a group of blind people were asked to describe the elephant standing in front of them, their answers depended on what part of the enormous creature was within arm's reach—"the rough, ropelike tail, the mighty, treelike legs, the twisting snake-like trunk," and so on. "Each blind man's version was wrong, but each possessed an element of the more complex elephantine truth."

However, when we look for life in interstellar space, it is impossible to agree with this position. And so NASA adopted "an agreed-upon definition of the term *life*." It is supposed to have three features. Firstly, it must be a system based on chemistry. And thus computer programs, robots activated by microprocessors and other, highly inventive electronic systems have no place in this definition. Secondly, life develops and maintains its existence by gathering both energy and atoms—from the surrounding environment, which is the essence of metabolism. And finally, the hallmark of life is changeability, without which evolution could not have been able to select more and more complex creatures. Armed with this definition, we set off in search of life beyond our planet.

Scientists accept that life began about four billion years ago on the youthful planet Earth. It grew out of primordial materials—air, water and rock. It was an example of emergence. This fashionable word defines how complex systems arise out of simple components, often in an unexpected way. This process supposedly proceeded according to the laws of physics and chemistry. From this point, agreement on the initial conditions and scenarios for the appearance of life on Earth diverge. For obvious reasons, the paleontologists train their sights on the oldest rocks. However, during their formation, these rocks were subjected to the effects of such extreme temperatures, pressures and gigantic distorting forces that they cannot possibly have preserved traces of life from that period inside them. Microscope examination, even based on analysis of the isotopes of coal and the decomposition of atomic spectrums, is not able to provide unambiguous answers. An example of this is the well-publicized recent scientific argument over whether one of the oldest rocks, which is 3.7 trillion years old, discovered in Australia (at the Apex Chert excavation site), conceals the image of primordial microbes. The people who noticed them have no doubt these are "the oldest, primordial bacteria." The skeptics, at an equally high scholarly level, do not hesitate to call this discovery a "Loch Ness monster." An apparently more certain method involves looking for bio-signatures, in other words, chemical compounds that are unambiguously produced solely by living organisms. They include polycyclic, five-ring hydrocarbons—hopanes—which are components of cell membranes. It was they that showed the presence of cyanobacteria—primitive microbes that feed the Earth's atmosphere with oxygen—in ancient, black, argillaceous slate. They are 2.7 trillion years old. And that is the record in the search for traces of life on Earth.

Meteorites are a source of undying fascination. Are they envoys from outer space that sowed life on Earth? Verifying this ever-current, hotly debated hypothesis comes up against some basic problems because of ... bacteria. Following its incredibly long journey, every meteorite has lain on Earth for at least a fortnight to many thousand years. Meanwhile, over a few months at most, bacteria have managed to get deep inside each meteorite through the tiniest chink. They seek sources of chemical energy, stored in the meteorite's minerals. Modern research documents a rich presence of bacteria in the most extreme environments: the eternal ice of the Antarctic, boiling geysers, the water in very acidic ponds, deep-sea hydro-thermal zones and the rock of the Earth's crust. So it is no surprise that the most famous meteorite is the one that fell on 28 September 1969 in a cow field near the village of Murchison, situated about a hundred miles from Melbourne in Australia. There were two reasons for its fame: it was large, containing over ten kilograms of rock. But the second reason was more important: "a number of pieces were collected while they were still warm." The chances of bacterial contamination were negligible. The first search for bio-signatures seemed positive, but the next one prompted doubts; they could have arisen in the extreme circumstances when the meteorite itself was formed. The riddle has yet to be resolved.

If we were to seek a place in the universe that is connected with life, nothing can compare with Mars. Its history began a hundred years ago, when the American astronomer Percival Lowell described a network of canals on the Red Planet, which in his opinion were proof of an advanced civilization. These fantastical visions fired the imaginations of science fiction writers for decades, and observations conducted by the Viking robot, which landed on Mars in the 1970s, providing ambiguous results, kept up the high temperature of debate. No solutions have resulted from modern research on the inside of a Martian meteorite either.

One thing remains: to construct life from the basics, in a test tube. The first step along this path was taken in 1951 by a young American postgraduate named Stanley Miller. After hearing a seminar by his supervisor, Harold Urey, on the origin of life on Earth, he gained his consent to change the subject of his doctoral thesis and set about preparing a famous experiment.

The setup for the experiment was simple and ingenious. It was "a primitive Earth sitting on a tabletop" inside two glass vessels. One vessel, filled with water and heated from the outside, reproduced a primitive ocean. The second, set higher, contained the ingredients of the Earth's early atmosphere: ammonia, methane and hydrogen. Electrodes were put inside the vessel holding the gases, ready to produce sparks in imitation of lightning. The "atmosphere," charged with electricity, was connected by an airtight pipe to the "ocean"; the entire arrangement was enclosed. After a few days of electrical discharges, new components began to collect in the "ocean": at least half a dozen amino acids and other organic molecules. And so in the primordial environment of Earth, chemical compounds that are the building blocks of life could come into being. The Miller-Urey experiment was an inspiration for many scientists. It was repeated hundreds, maybe thousands of times, with modifications of the combination of gases, the water temperature, pressure and so on, and every time it produced all manner of organic compounds. As the years passed however, criticisms were voiced. The composition of gases was questioned. It seems that the primordial atmosphere did not contain methane or ammonia, but other, less reactive ingredients, from which it would have been much harder to obtain organic compounds. In addition, and this was the most important complaint, the primitive ocean, known as "primordial or prebiotic soup," was an incredibly diluted solution; the likelihood of a reaction between two molecules was negligible. This problem is well known in medicine and concerns clotting of the blood. For blood to clot, a number of proteins that circulate in the blood must inter-react. But if, for example, they were to meet at the site of a wound and start to react with each other, we would have enough time to bleed to death before coagulation took place. In reality, some small blood cells called thrombocytes are aroused and drag these clotting proteins to their surfaces. Once concentrated there, they act like lightning: the reaction to produce the end product (thrombin) happens 300,000 times faster and the blood clots instantly.

A surface of this kind, where amino acids scattered about the primordial ocean would have met and concentrated, could have been provided by the ubiquitous mineral pyrite, also known as iron sulfide. So says a brilliant theory developed by Günter

Wächtershäuser. The mineral would have created a skeleton, a support, on which organic particles would have settled and started an exchange of their products, in other words, metabolism. Otherwise, the products made would be irrevocably lost in the depths of the primordial ocean. This bold concept, once called heretical, has firm chemical foundations. It does not take much to demonstrate experimentally that the major cycle of biochemical transformations in animals and in people, known as the Krebs cycle, can happen on the catalytic surface of pyrite. It would have been a flat world, a very thin, single layer of self-replicating molecules covering in an invisible membrane a firm base made of iron and sulfur. Such a world could have lasted for eons, resistant to the effect of an environment that would have killed living cells.

However, those who believe that first RNA had to come into being, and that metabolism only appeared after it, follow the research of Swiss chemist Albert Eschenmoser. He synthesized nucleic acids from simpler sugars than the ones that form DNA and RNA, namely from four-carbon carbohydrates, or tetroses. The molecules obtained in this way, although simpler than RNA, are strikingly similar to it and can cast some light on the mysteries of its origin. Finally, some physicists, immersed in their own world, suggest radically different solutions. Let us drop the remote idea, they say, that organic chemistry explains the origin of life. It offers no kind of bridge between inanimate and animate matter. Let us stop babbling about prebiotic soup. It "could be that quantum mechanics enabled life to emerge directly from the atomic world, without the need for complex intermediate chemistry." Information can be recreated at the quantum level, in the simplest replicator, thousands of times faster than in a modern computer. It can be passive—using, for example, the orientation of the spin of an electron and such useful phenomena as "entanglement," "superposition" and "tunneling." However, no one knows where to look for the quantum replicator that is once supposed to have started life. Certainly not in the by-now-traditional "prebiotic soup." Maybe in icy interstellar space? Wherever it might be, the replicators of information, once established, would have at their disposal built-in variability and diversity, in accordance with Heisenberg's uncertainty principle, which would be the foundation of Darwinian evolution. And at a certain stage, quantum life could turn to organic particles to support and strengthen its memory. This sort of vision leads us to the astrobiologists' burning question: was the start of life a pure accident, or the expected result of physical laws conducive to its development? And to a further, existential question: is life a universal phenomenon, or are we alone in the boundless universe?

After these cosmic perspectives, it is worth listening to the voice of some sober philosophers who compare our feverish "attempts to define life with similar eighteenth-century efforts to characterize water." At the time water's purity and wetness were raised, its capacity to maintain life, to freeze at a low temperature and to flow downhill on sloping ground, as well as many other features that, even when combined, were not sufficient or necessary. None of these definitions could capture the essence of water, which was only brought by atomic theory: molecules consisting of two hydrogen atoms and one oxygen atom. At the start of the twenty-first century, science finds itself in a similar situation. Without familiarity with the fundamental laws of biology, which probably do exist, although they are hidden from us, we will never catch the definition of life in a net of concepts. If it ever does happen, the question of whether viruses are alive or not will cease to be a riddle without an answer.

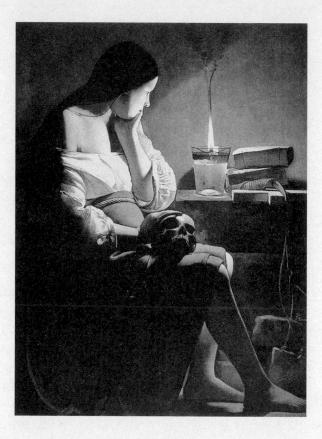

Georges de la Tour
Magdalen with the Smoking Flame, c. 1640
Los Angeles County Museum of Art

ON DYING AND DEATH

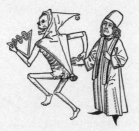

"Don't you think I'm an anomaly of nature?" Czesław Miłosz asked me when he reached the end of his ninety-second year of life. And it occurred to me that he was like a mighty Lithuanian oak tree, its leaves rustling with poetry. His mind, supported by a memory I have never known anyone else to have, tried more and more often to fathom the essence of illness, and also death. It never seemed to rest at all, except during sleep, which sometimes lasted longer because of illness. Once, after several days of deep unconsciousness, as soon as he came to, he said a brief thank-you and at once added: "A new book absolutely has to be written about dying and death." "A sort of modern version of the *Ars moriendi*, transferred from the Middle Ages?" I asked. "Would anyone want to read it?" He had no doubts about that. He knew he would not have time to write the book himself. In any case, he reckoned a doctor should do it, to show how we undergo this final test, describe the process of dying and the ways in which death comes upon us and achieves its end.

"But there are a thousand ways to die" (*Occurrunt animo*

pereundi mille figurae), said Ariadne when Theseus deserted her. This foreigner, whom she had helped to kill her bull-headed step-brother the Minotaur, for whom she ran away from the royal palace and whose feet she was willing to wash in Athens like a common serving maid, left her on a wild, rocky island, which became once and for all "the landscape of rejected love." As she spoke these words from a clifftop by the sea, was she thinking of her magnificent, shameless mother, Queen Pasiphaë, and her sister Phedra, wracked by pangs of conscience, both of them overwhelmed by the bewitching power of love, which drove them to suicide? Did she already know she was destined for the same fate too? A violent death, which by its sudden and unexpected nature shocks the victim's loved ones and everyone around them, and brings a pain that can only be compared with the despair of a mother when she loses the child she is expecting before it is born? Sudden death, which Hippocrates called apoplexy, explained as "striking one down like a thunderbolt," is present today, just like thousands of years ago, whether self-inflicted or caused by someone else, by a disease affecting the heart or the brain, a traffic accident, a tsunami or the collapsing roof of a covered market. We always fear it, and we can hear an echo of that fear in the Catholic prayer: "Deliver us, O Lord, from a sudden and unprovided death." In my childhood years, before the Second Vatican Council, in the days of the Latin liturgy, sudden death had the face of the Normans. So, quite unwittingly, we were still issuing a collective imprecation from centuries ago, praying for God to avert their furious advance and save us from the *furor Normanorum*. Invaders from the north attacked suddenly, bringing death and leaving nothing:

> *An immense coldness from the Longobards*
> *Their shadow sears the grass when they flock into the valley*
> *Shouting their protracted nothingnothingnothing*

There are still plenty of descendants of the Longobards around, but in his everyday practice the doctor encounters sudden death in illness: in heart attacks, strokes and poisoning, and after road accidents. Immediate resuscitation can often bring the patient back to life. But if it is performed with a few minutes' delay, even though the heart starts to beat again and the lungs to respire, consciousness does not return. The family and the doctor wait in hope, counting the days and then the weeks, but the patient does not awake from his coma. And so belated resuscitation transfers the rescued person to another state of existence, unknown to mankind in our entire history. This is *vita vegetativa*. Do these patients really live the life of plants? Because they remain rooted to a single spot without moving away from us or coming towards us, and without reacting? They lie in hospitals, hospices or at home, suspended between life and death. They do not react to external stimuli. They are fed through tubes inserted into the stomach. They make grunting sounds and sometimes they move a hand or open their eyes, but their gaze remains empty. They have extensive damage on both sides of the cerebral cortex, although the structures of the brain stem remain intact. They really are alive; no one doubts it — they are on the same side as we are. So we try to make contact with them, if only the merest hint of it. We are on the alert, like wireless operators waiting to hear if something will break through all the buzzing and crackling in the headphones. The patient's loved ones try to get through to him, wherever he is, and give him a sign that he has not been abandoned, to show they are still with him. They squeeze his hand, adapt the rhythm of their own breathing to his and whisper stories of everyday life into his ear in an effort to transfer him into it. It is like sending signals into outer space in search of extraterrestrial civilizations, and just as hard to get an answer. And when we see a mother remaining with her child who is in a coma, not for months but for years, out of what the poet Cyprian Norwid called "fellow feeling," in other words, a feeling shared with the patient, it occurs to us that perhaps "life involves maturing to the awareness that it is all about being dedicated to others."

In situations of this kind we cannot avoid the question of limit. For how long should this other state of existence be artificially sustained? This question went around the world in the case of Terri Schiavo, the forty-year-old American woman who in early youth, for reasons that cannot be fully explained, suffered cardiac arrest and underwent clinical death, but was resuscitated after a ten-minute delay. For the next fifteen years she was in a deep coma, completely out of touch, although her heart was beating and she was breathing. Her life was kept going by sustenance fed to her intravenously. Finally her husband made a decision, in defiance of her parents' wishes, and the federal courts confirmed it. Her drip was disconnected, and Terri died ten days later, on 30 March 2005. Who really has to decide in such situations? The spouse? The court? The parents? In fact it is usually the mute decision of the doctors.

But some doctors believe that in a flooded brain some islands may have survived that show traces of life. And they try to get through to them. When the observations made by some British neurologists in the case of a twenty-three-year-old woman were published in fall 2006, they caused quite a stir. Five months after an accident, the patient was in a coma and fulfilled all the criteria for a vegetative state. When this deeply unconscious person was told to imagine she was "playing a game of tennis," and another time that she was "visiting all of the rooms of her house," signs of activity appeared in her brain in two areas, different from each other, but corresponding to ones that in many healthy people are activated after the same instructions. These islands lit up on the screens of a functional MRI, testifying to increased consumption of oxygen by the cerebral tissue. However, the skeptics are not convinced that they were the regions of the brain "necessary or sufficient for performing" these tasks. It is also claimed that the patient may already have entered the first stage of improvement, which was evident several months later. Either way, the definition of the vegetative state may be questioned in the not-too-distant future.

This is also implied by the story of a thirty-nine-year-old man who, after a serious motorcycle accident, spent nineteen years in a state of so-called minimal consciousness, which means that he sporadically reacted to a voice by moving his head, but could not communicate either by gesture or word. In 2003, in the course of a few months, he regained the power of speech, and ultra-sensitive examination revealed that "neurons in his brain had been slowly reconnecting over the years to bypass damaged regions." Need I add that the first word to emerge from the lips of the patient after almost twenty years was "Mom"?!

For thousands of years, medicine used the classic criteria for death: cessation of circulation and breathing. When the blood stopped circulating, the dead person's body went cold, livid spots (*livor mortis*) appeared and finally rigor mortis set in. These were the irreversible hallmarks, and the only thing left to consider was the funeral. The spread in the 1960s of resuscitation and the use of respirators revealed the inadequacy of these criteria for death. Indeed, in many cases the circulation and breathing could be restored; clinical death had become reversible. The brain and its ways of dying then found themselves at the center of interest. A new criterion for death was formulated: irreversible, permanent cessation of brain function. Particular attention was paid to the brain stem, and we began to identify the life of the brain stem directly with the life of the entire brain, and indirectly with the life of the organism as a whole.

The stem is the structure that links the brain to the spinal cord. It houses the centers that control breathing, the working of the heart and muscles, blood vessel tension and coordination of eyeball movements. Nerve paths run through the stem to the cerebral cortex from all parts of the body and go back to them through the stem too, though along different routes. Here too is the "reticular substance" (*substantia reticularis*), which turns on the cerebral cortex and maintains its state of wakefulness and awareness. How does a doctor seek symptoms of the death of the brain stem? He shines a light in the eyes and confirms that the pupils are failing to react, touches the eyeball and sees that the eyelids are not blinking, presses the trigeminal nerve in the face to cause pain but gets no response and moves the breathing tube but fails to prompt a reflex cough. He performs all these simple tests and several others at least in order to check if there is still a flicker of life in some hidden corner of the brain. He repeats them three or six hours later, and if the result is just as negative, he diagnoses death and recognizes the patient as deceased. And so he establishes the diagnosis by doing some relatively simple tests, without any sophisticated equipment; in many countries, including Poland, not even an electroencephalogram is required, because it is not fully reliable. In the modern understanding, death takes some time to occur. It is not a single moment, but a complex process. A person dies in stages: first biologically, when the brain stem dies. The remaining organs and groups of cells die later, each in its own time.

The definition in which brain death means the death of the organism as a whole has been adopted by most countries. Yet it still stirs emotions and objections. Let us think what a family experiences when they come into contact with a loved one who has been declared dead according to the new criterion for death. The loved one's body bears no signs of death: it is warm, it is breathing, the heart is beating and the blood is circulating. "If the sick or dying person looks exactly the same today as he did yesterday, why is he being treated as if he were alive yesterday but dead today? Can the pronouncement of death have no connection with the experience of death?" Naturally, among the critics we hear voices saying that brain death has been invented for the needs of transplant surgery. The complexity of the problem is revealed by the debate about Terri Schiavo. To this day some leading authorities believe that the changes in her were not irreversible; she was breathing on her own and her brain stem was functioning. "But in spite of that the decision was taken to starve her to death, because the law allowed it."

For us, the doctors, turning off a respirator is an admission of failure. Deep in our hearts, each of us deludes himself that maybe in just a little more time, just a few days, maybe the organism will get moving. But you cannot go on like that ad infinitum. Hence the need for objective criteria that dispel the doubts and avoid the insoluble situation in which the quantum physicists found themselves with Schrödinger's cat—half dead and half alive.

One might think resuscitation came into being only in the lifetime of the last generation; certainly, in that time it has become available publicly and on a large scale. But in fact it has its roots in the dawn of medicine. It was for this, for resurrecting the dead, that Asclepius, the god of medicine, was struck down with a thunderbolt. Later on, the idea of "reanimation" was always recurring in dreams and fantasies about loved ones who were lost and gone. It accompanied doctors and charlatans seeking applause and fame. It also attracted the imagination of painters, and not surprisingly, Caravaggio could not resist it. He painted his picture *The Raising of Lazarus* in the final period of his life, when after escaping from prison on the island of Malta by letting himself down its precipitous walls on a rope straight into the sea, he got across the bay and reached Sicily. In Messina he received a commission from a rich Genoese merchant called Giovanni Battista de Lazzari. The painting made reference to the merchant's name and was destined for the altar in the chapel of a hospital brotherhood caring for the sick. Caravaggio, the greatest painter in Italy, accepted a huge fee in advance and was given the hospital's best rooms as his studio. He worked in secret, and made the workmen posing for him hold up a corpse that was already in a state of decay, and that served him as the model for Lazarus. The picture amazed the citizens of Messina, who expressed certain reservations. Enraged by their provincial complaints, Caravaggio ripped the painting to shreds with a stiletto. Once he had calmed down, he painted a second one, and this version has survived.

The story of Lazarus is told to us in the Gospel of Saint John. He was dying in Bethany, and his sisters sent for Jesus, but when the Savior arrived, He found Lazarus had already been lying in his grave for four days. He ordered the stone covering the tomb to be moved aside and called out in a loud voice. And the dead man came out with his hands and feet bandaged. Caravaggio's Lazarus is getting up with great difficulty; his transparently painted body is still rigid with rigor mortis, and only his right hand is opening to accept Christ's light. His outstretched arms herald the crucifixion. His body remains torn between light and shadow. The picture, as envisaged for the hospital chapel, shows the struggle between life and death and the hope for atonement. It has feverish, apocalyptic overtones: in it the "desperate longing for grace, the terror of the dreams that may disturb the sleep of death" are striking. Shimmering with reflections, the paint seems to correspond to the artist's state of agitation. It is said that one day during a break in work on *The Raising of Lazarus*, Caravaggio went into the nearby church of the Madonna del Piero. There he was offered holy water to wash away his everyday sins. "It is not necessary," he replied, "since all my sins are mortal."

Caravaggio was no exception. Other master painters too sometimes painted death from nature, by looking at corpses, even obtained for a single night. But, of course, they could never compare in number with all the doctors who from Renaissance times onwards sought dead bodies in order to investigate the obscurities hidden by layers of flesh and open up the world locked inside us — in short, to perform postmortems. William Harvey, who discovered the mystery of blood circulation, personally performed autopsies on his own father and sister, not to mention his wife's beloved canary. As he said himself, he had no choice. Never for a moment did he consider stopping his scientific research, and he had no intention of stealing corpses from the graveyard. However, this was a practice that was already common in his lifetime, in seventeenth-century England, and that would become extremely widespread over the next one hundred and fifty years, because the law threatened severe punishments for stealing valuables from tombs, but not dead bodies. Teachers of medicine encouraged their apprentices in the medical art to obtain corpses for practical studies. Records have survived saying that at some Scottish medical schools, tuition fees could be paid in bodies instead of money. At the London academies, demand grew so rapidly that a clan of body hunters came into being. In a document issued by the House of Commons in 1828, we read that a gang consisting of six "resurrectionists," as they were called, had dug up three hundred and twelve bodies in the academic season, in other words, from October to May, earning one thousand pounds a year, which was several times more than an unqualified workman earned. And in addition, the document states, they had the whole summer off.

Professional grave robbers stole thousands of corpses from their tombs for Doctor John Hunter, a Scot, the most famous surgeon in eighteenth-century London, whom the British like to call "the father of modern surgery." He dissected all the dead bodies obtained for him and made some original observations in the fields of anatomy and embryology. An ardent supporter of experimentation, he told his pupil Edward Jenner, who discovered the inoculation for smallpox: "I think your solution is just, but why think? Why not try the experiment?" He was not puffed up with pride, but could see the limitations of his profession, and left us the following definition of a surgeon: "An armed savage who attempts to get that by force which a civilized man would get by stratagem." But this sober man with his feet fixed firmly on the ground was overcome by desire. He longed to possess the body of the famous Irish giant, Charles Byrne, who was dying of consumption. He sent his lackeys after him, who pursued him day and night, waiting for him to die. The terrified giant drew up a will in which he gave instructions for his body to be sunk in the Irish Sea. Hunter spent a fortune to bribe the undertaker, who at a roadside tavern on the way to the sea, extracted the corpse from the coffin and replaced it with cobblestones, while the mourners, who were extremely drunk, were fast asleep. And so the great surgeon's dream came true.

Let us remember Rembrandt's painting, *The Anatomy Lesson of Professor Tulp*, featuring the grandeur of death, and the concentration and awe of the doctors faced with the mysteries of the human body. Taking part in an autopsy was in those days regarded as such a distinction that the names of those present are written on a piece of paper being held in the picture by one of the men gathered around Professor Tulp; they have survived to the present day. However, once dissections had become a common affair, their image changed too. In 1828 the young Hector Berlioz assisted at a postmortem and left a description of it in his diary. He was shocked by the sight of the floor covered in puddles of blood and scattered bones, with rats roaming among them. We shall spare the Reader further details of his description, from which it is easy to understand why the young man chose music and not medicine. But even Doctor Robert White, the eminent American neurosurgeon, who is the only man to have transplanted the heads of chimpanzees, told me in 2004: "I have never dared show anyone the film of that experiment. It was such a bloodbath!"

As for modern anatomy lessons … You might think we are light years away from Rembrandt. It is the year 2003; let us transport ourselves to the Atlantis Gallery in London. Outside there is a very long queue of people waiting to go in. Every day, thousands of the living file past the dead, who have been preserved far from here, in Dalian, a northern province of China. There, in mighty bunkers, two hundred Chinese are busy removing the skin from the human bodies sent from all corners of the Earth, taking months to prepare them so that millions of people worldwide can "see what's under your hood." The mummification technique was invented by German anatomist Gunther von Hagens. They call him "the Walt Disney of Death," although he prefers to say of himself that he simply reveals the beauty hidden under the skin. He dehydrates the corpses with ice-cold acetone and then injects them with synthetic polymers, plastic. The organs and tissues keep their build, right down to microscopic structures.

In the gallery the crowd walks among the "plastinates," which are displayed in various poses. But we are not at a waxworks exhibition. The plastinates are not imitating people. They are people, dead ones. One of them, stripped of his skin, is holding it like a jacket over his arm; he looks like a figure from Michelangelo's *Last Judgment*. Others are standing or sitting in relaxed poses. Besides the "full human specimens," there are some separate exhibits including a pair of tobacco-blackened lungs, a liver eaten away by cancer and a heart destroyed by an infarction. The visitors inspect them with curiosity. Do they also feel a shudder? More like a tickle, as here in the gallery you can hear occasional bursts of laughter and jovial comments. Before the Londoners, millions of people in New York and Munich came to see the plastinates. The exhibition is touring the world. In Korea the crowds came flocking day and night, and they had to keep the doors open round the clock to accommodate more than two-and-a-half million people. All over the world, the reactions are positive. Almost five thousand of the visitors have expressed a wish to be plastinated too.

The multiplied nature of the exhibition is a reflection of our world. Everything has been multiplied in this modern, mass anatomy lesson. Instead of a small group of students, leaning over a single corpse, hundreds of people are walking about among dozens of exposed bodies. Is it exhibitionism? All just for show? Many people believe these are features of our world. In the modern postutopian discourse, writes Chantal Delsol, "one major idea dominates . . . : the certainty, clung to come hell or high water, that man is indeterminate, thus preserving our liberty to do with him what we will. Man must be empty and malleable, capable of becoming anything." Thoughts about departing this life and the threat of death, seen face-to-face, have been left far behind. Rest in plastic, Reader!

Fifty, one hundred, five hundred years ago, those who departed this life did not have to be sought in museums. The dead came out to meet us themselves. So it was during the summer holidays of my childhood that I spent in Pilzno, my father's small native town in the Carpathian foothills. The local train, known as the "Bummelzug," panting away, would stop at the empty little station in Czarna. There the horses in harness would already be waiting to take us, our parents and all our holiday luggage home through the dark woods along a rutted sandy track. Whenever I read Mickiewicz's epic *Pan Tadeusz*, it is this white, stone quasi-manor house with a wooden veranda and a large garden that always springs to mind as soon as the hero's estate, Soplicowo, is mentioned. On hot summer afternoons, when life was at a standstill and the heat came wafting all the way from the Ukrainian steppes, the bells of the parish church and the monastery would ring out. After a brief jangling, the swinging tones would fall into a steady rhythm, and a funeral cortège would emerge from the parish church, cross the town's market square and go up Węgierska Street. It would pass under our windows on its way to the cemetery, which lay on a hill among old oak trees and poplars; through them in the distance we could see the river glinting and the outline of the mountains. At the front walked a peasant in too short a surplice, holding upright, in both hands, a long cross, taller than himself. Then came the coffin, on a horse-drawn hearse, though sometimes the relatives carried it on their shoulders. Next came the priest in his stole, holding a missal and a sprinkler, and behind him came the procession of people in black. Many years later we carried my father along this same route. The bells rang steadily and the singing of the mourners carried a long way. Ever since, I have heard these two bells, from the parish church and the monastery, in the funeral march out of Chopin's sonata in B-minor. They rang in two chords *basso ostinato*, relentlessly repeated, as the dotted, melodious tune unrolled above them.

These days, the town no longer comes out en masse to bid farewell to the deceased. No cortège crosses it, and no bells ring. From a chapel in a new part of the cemetery the coffin emerges on the platform of an electric trolley, on which it travels to the spot prepared for it in a long line of confusingly similar graves.

For centuries death communed with a man for a long time before taking him away. It accompanied him in his thoughts, conversations and prayers. In the fifteenth century didactic poems, such as *The Plaint of the Dying*, for example, were meant to "encourage a person to be pious, make him abhor sin, and instill in his heart a fear of death without repentance." The most successful of them, and "of all medieval Polish poetry in general," was *Master Polikarp's Conversation with Death*. At his request, Death appears in a church to a learned man named Master Polikarp. The Master faints, regains consciousness and starts up a conversation with Death. He asks about its origin, and it replies that it was born in Paradise, when Eve plucked the apple: "Adam tempted me with the apple." Angry and ironical, Death unfurls its vision of omnipotence and might. Then the Master timidly asks why we have doctors. In reply he hears: "Every doctor's a cheating fraud; none of his ointments do any good." And to dispel any doubts, he adds:

> *There's no escaping from my scythe*
> *I slash the throat of all who live.*

In our poem about Master Polikarp, Death was depicted as a decaying corpse; this element of horror was not at all exceptional in those days. However, the personification of death that prevailed was not known to the ancient world or in the early Middle Ages — in this version it was embodied as a skeleton. Especially popular in painting and in fairground shows was the *danse macabre*, or *Totentanz*. It expressed the medieval concept of human life, where everyone is equal, heading towards death. Death leads the dance, in which people of every age and status take part, including a pope, an emperor, a cardinal, some bishops, a girl and a child. In the Bernardine church in Krakow a fiddler and an organist with a small harmonium play along to some skeletons dancing a quadrille. Death has one paw resting on the fiddler's shoulder and is holding the organist around the waist, while politely holding up his notes. A caption under one of the dance scenes assures us that "what a dreadful leap up high, when the tune screams you must die."

The presence of the dead weighs heavy on the Middle Ages, both in the real and the imagined world. From the tenth century onwards, stories about ghosts that torment the living are heard everywhere. These ghosts are usually the phantoms of people who died violently—murder victims, women in childbirth, unbaptized babies and suicides. They demand support from the living—alms and prayers—which will allow them to escape hell. Sometimes the phantoms emerge from their graves, attack the living and drink their blood. In the word "macabre" some historians have noticed an onomatopoeia, hearing "the rattle of bones," while others have interpreted it as "the dance of the spindleshanks" (*mactorum chorea*). The whole art of the macabre—the iconography, frescoes, sculptures, miniatures and etchings—shocks the mind with the threat of death. In contrast to our era, where fear focuses on the pain of dying, in medieval times the greatest fear was prompted by sudden death. It carried the danger of departing this life in a state of mortal sin, and thus increased the threat of damnation in hell. Only the eighteenth century brings a third place, a waiting room for ordinary sinners—purgatory.

Did its omnipresence in the Middle Ages mean that death had become something tame and familiar? Was it less bitter and cruel than nowadays? This is a marked contrast to the modern attitude, in which we do our best to forget about death—we have driven it out of our world. "Death is a scandal, just like pain and suffering." But in his extraordinary, pioneering book *The Waning of the Middle Ages*, Johan Huizinga reckons that when the world was over five hundred years younger, all forms of human life had far sharper contours than they do today. "The contrast between suffering and joy, between adversity and happiness, appeared more striking. All experience had yet to the minds of men the directness and absoluteness of the pleasure and pain of child-life." There can be no doubt that in the Middle Ages people spoke more sincerely and commonly about dying and death than today, which does not mean it was any calmer a process.

These matters cannot be generalized, just like the trauma of the death of a loved one and our reactions to their death, which the hospital doctor sees every day. Often it is a silent grief, a torpor, a desire to get away from the place of suffering, a speedy farewell — especially when the illness has gone on for a long time, chronically. But a great many people are dumbstruck at the news of sudden, unexpected death. Their expression goes blank and they fall silent, as if "tongue-tied," while in fact they are in the grip of some powerful emotions that have shattered their peace. This sort of situation is described by the myth of Niobe, who after the death of her children freezes on the spot and turns to stone. Another response to the news of the death of a loved one is fainting — terrifying fear of an extreme situation that cannot be altered. Keeping calm and still can at any moment turn into an outburst of spasmodic pain. "We would recall the irrevocable; we would cry out to one who cannot answer; we beg for the touch of a hand whose loving pressure we shall never feel again." Joanna, the sixteenth-century Queen of Castile, known as the Mad, twice had her husband's coffin opened at Miraflores where he was buried. According to some accounts, she tore the clothing from him, kissing his feet and hands; others say that she stood motionless, without shedding a single tear. One of the most famous examples of long-term mourning in history is the case of the British queen Victoria over the loss of her beloved husband, Albert. Even though in time she managed to overcome her initial state of depression, she could not control her extravagant grief. She always dressed in black; imposed a strict cult of the deceased, celebrating the anniversaries of his birth and death and the dates of their engagement and marriage; had Albert's rooms kept in an unaltered state and for a long time failed to observe mourning for any other member of the family. So is it true to say that "in all these strivings of ours to keep the dead from really being so, we begin to encompass their real extinction within us"?

In the German language, as in ancient Greece, death (*der Tod*) is of the masculine gender. In the first of three drawings by Albrecht Dürer, known as masterpieces, Death and the Devil never abandon the knight in armor, who resembles an equestrian statue in bronze. In Paul Celan's most famous lyric poem, *Todesfuge* — "The Fugue of Death" — "'Death is a master from Germany' and is embodied in the figure of a man playing with snakes; he has blue eyes and forces the Jews to dance. 'In German art, from Holbein's to Rethlowski's *Dance of Death*, death remains an aggressive, active, vigorous man, sometimes in armor, sometimes on a horse.'"

In the Polish language, this association is not made because death (*śmierć*) is of the feminine gender and has a woman's face. Jacek Malczewski painted her many times over a twenty-year period, and no other theme appears so consistently in his work. Nor does any other more powerfully depict the tension between the biological and the transient. In his painting *Death*, dated 1917, a strong, healthy looking girl stands by the smooth white wall of a cottage. She has black, slicked-back hair with a flower pinned in it and is wearing a simple, deep purple dress tied at the waist. She is waiting by an open window, in which we can see the face of an old man. Leaning against her shoulder there is a scythe, "painted with tangible precision." She has turned her head towards the open window. In her there is strength, physicality, beauty and indifference. "She is young — so she has time to wait . . . , she is healthy — so she conquers even the healthiest."

In another painting a naked woman of luxuriant physical beauty invites an old man to come through the gate, beyond which there is no return. Another especially eloquent painting is *Death*, dated 1902. A young woman reaper is wielding a scythe, and an old man has knelt down and folded his hands in prayer, accepting the light but attentive touch of her fingers on his eyelids as a revelation. This sort of image of death — gentle and feminine — seems to imply being reconciled with fate. There is nothing off-putting or threatening here. The picture radiates extraordinary charm, emanating benevolence, tranquility and solace. Death by touch soothes the pain, betokens another life and promises "unity with whatever man loved most ardently in life."

The mood for crossing to the other side in silence and solace is set — as well as by profound faith — by old age. The time when "the clocks began to turn / faster and faster above us." Ever more frequent signals appear telling us that ". . . the whole thing must oxidise, / disintegrate and cool, turn pabulum." For ages we do our best to resist them: "Each night, each day the tiresome exercise / so no small change should change the enterprise." But it is late already. We cannot hold back the changes forever. And so we start to move away from life. We stop expecting anything, either good or bad, and nothing unusual or surprising is likely to happen any more. Man ages gradually; first his curiosity about people and the world wanes. Gradually, it all becomes familiar and obvious, and things lose their mystery. At the same time the body grows older — not the whole thing, not all at once, but in parts. The vision and hearing grow weaker, and the heart or lungs deteriorate. A sort of worm seems to be gnawing away at us. Our physical powers diminish and tiredness sets in. Every outing from home becomes a problem and assumes the proportions of a major event. Meanwhile, hope remains alive within us, the desire for change and even joy. But once they too have gone and there is nothing left except memory and vanity, then old age takes possession of us for good and all. We just continue to watch over the body, the fabric that keeps disintegrating faster and faster, irreversibly. Along with old age, death starts to creep in. Things that were never going to concern us come closer and make a lair for themselves inside us. Death blends in, "She is a body in your body. . . . She swells in you, rots like an alder trunk felled into water." The rotting stump becomes more and more of a burden. Frightened, confused signals run round the body and reach the brain. It tries to stifle them, until gradually it slides into depression. Death does not come from the outside. It is inside us. One day "we find it, like something that is found in the pocket of a winter coat."

If the circle of life heads towards its close by bringing us via old age — that "second childishness" — back to the beginning, then death goes even further, reaches back even earlier and, in marking the limit of life, evokes the first moments of our existence. For it is then, paradoxically, that it makes its very first appearance within us. In embryonic life, inside the mother's womb, some of the fetus's cells grow, but others perish. Their death does not happen by accident, but is carefully prepared, planned in advance. Most of the cells in adult human beings preserve from that remote time a precise mechanism for suicidal destruction. It is built into their structure and is called apoptosis. When the right signal comes through, the cell goes into a lethal trajectory. And like an intercontinental missile, it is steered by a program that has been prerecorded in minute detail, and that has just one aim: annihilation and self-destruction. A network of specialized enzymes is set in motion, called caspases, which disjoint the cell into "pure," defined pieces without stimulating the inflammatory reaction that always accompanies its unforeseen damage and disintegration. So, for example, in early fetal life, to begin with our fingers are fused together, but they separate when the cells joining them enter into apoptosis and die.

However, in waterbirds they remain alive, creating web footing. It is also thanks to apoptosis in the early stages of life that the thymus eliminates autoreactive lymphocytes, instructing the immune system how to distinguish the "self" from the "non-self." A cell in which the apoptosis mechanism has once been set in motion goes on a journey from which there is no return, heading for the same goal as an old person, for whom we cannot restrain the process of dying.

When Seamus Heaney, the great poet and Nobel Prize winner, visited Czesław Miłosz a few months before his death, he found him in the sitting room, face-to-face with a bronze bust of Carol, his second wife who had died a year earlier. Heaney got the impression that the old poet sitting on the far side of the room was staring at the bronze bust and everything else from another shore. Around him were his daughter-in-law, our two best nurses and, in the background, his invaluable housekeeper and his secretary. All this vigilant care and his host's altered expression made Heaney think of Oedipus, nursed by his daughters in a grove at Colonus. The old king had come to the place where, as he knew, his life would end. For Miłosz, Krakow was not his native city, but it was there, like Oedipus at Colonus, that "he had come home to himself, to the world, and to the otherworld." Here for the whole eighth decade of his life and the years that followed, he was living testimony to Goethe's words about the potential that remains in old age, about the fact that "it does not have to be nothing but decay, but can also be *Steigerung*, a heightening." When, less than a year after this final visit, Heaney flew to Miłosz's funeral, he brought his own adaptation of an extract from Sophocles's *Oedipus at Colonus*. In it, as he bids his daughters farewell, Oedipus takes them into his arms and says:

... "My children," he said —
And the rest of us felt that we were his then too —
"Today is the day that ends your father's life.
The burden I have been to myself and you
Is lifted. And yet it was eased by love.
Now you must do without me and relearn
The meaning of that word by remembering."

Sometimes a person does not know life has already started to escape him "like grains of sand pouring through a sieve." He comes to see the doctor with some fairly trivial complaint, but the examination reveals the unexpected truth: the *signum mali omnis* — a sentence against which there is no appeal. A portent of life's end can also reach us by a different route, as it did Homer. One day, he was walking along the beach when he stopped by a boat, from which some young fishermen were unloading their catch. "How did you do, boys?" he asked. The youngest one replied with a riddle: "All that we caught, we left in the sea; all that we did not catch, we are taking home with us." Then Homer remembered the words of the Delphic oracle, warning him against boys talking in riddles. He did not understand what the youth's reply meant, but he did realize that the end of his life had come. He died three days later. However, what the fishermen were thinking of was fleas. Any that they caught on themselves, they threw into the sea, but of course any that they did not catch, they brought home with them. No account has survived of the last three days of Homer, who was himself one great enigma. However, we have no reason to suppose he did not show the same *areté* — courage determining perfection — as his compatriot Socrates did hundreds of years later, the man who the Delphic oracle would say was the wisest of the Greeks.

He could easily have avoided death, but he refused to do so, and insisted on obeying the law. To the very end he talked with his pupils and accepted death with exemplary calm and bravery. "Everyone unanimously admits that no man before, as far back as our memory reaches, ever looked in the eyes of death with greater dignity," wrote his pupil Xenophon. Socrates was the son of a midwife, who understood that the truth *arises* among questions, and who called the method of reaching the truth that he created *maieutics*, or the art of obstetrics. He believed that the truth is inside us, though we are usually unaware of it. He aimed to bring out of hiding, into the light of day, some invariable truths and fundamental ideas, mainly concerning morality. Before his death he turned his thoughts to medicine. His last words were: "Crito, we ought to offer a cock to Asclepius. See to it, and don't forget." His enigmatic words, still discussed at length, are interpreted in various ways. Was this his way of saying that to live means to be ill for a long time, and so we should thank Asclepius for postponing the end? No one has offered a more radical interpretation than Friedrich Nietzsche, who wrote: "Socrates *wanted* to die ... He forced Athens to sentence him ... ; he said softly to himself ... 'Socrates himself has merely been sick a long time.'" But it is hard to regard Nietzsche's judgment as impartial. Indeed, after discerning with astonishing perspicacity the wave of European nihilism heralding "the death of God," he was looking for its genesis and perceived it ... even in Socrates's rationalist dialectics. Yet he admired him for his death: "To die proudly when it is no longer possible to live proudly." And he was probably thinking of Socrates when he wrote appreciatively about freely chosen death as "death at the right time, brightly and cheerfully accomplished amid children and witnesses: then a real farewell is still possible, as the one who is taking leave is still there."

Socrates's last words, uttered while fully conscious, have come down to us unchanged. However, the doctor's mind has a right to be doubtful when he reads about words spoken in the final throes of death. We find the first version of Słowacki's last words, spoken on his deathbed shortly after listening to a letter from his mother, in a letter written by his friend Zygmunt Szczęsny Feliński the day after his death. The poet spent his final hours dictating to Feliński corrections to the second rhapsody in *King-Spirit*, and then finally asked to be laid on the pillows in his bed and was supposed to have said: "Maybe it will be in this position that death will find me." But a dozen years later Feliński, then a senior church hierarch, made these words sound more impressive; others then "worked some more on the phrase," which in the ultimate version was to be: "The time has come to cast off this tattered mantle." Yet Słowacki died suffocating. Terrible attacks of breathlessness and coughing interrupted by fainting fits came one after another, without any respite towards the end. His words must have been mixed with whistling and wheezing, and it was probably very hard for them, especially the final ones, to break through his airways once they were blocked.

Do dying people see visions in their death throes, and of whom? Does anyone come for them? We can only make guesses, as did Giuseppe Tomasi di Lampedusa. As Prince Fabrizio, the keen amateur astronomer, was dying, his mind was plunged in darkness and he kept losing consciousness. It seemed to him as if, with a small group of relatives surrounding his deathbed, "suddenly amid the group appeared a young woman; slim, in brown traveling dress and wide bustle, with a straw hat trimmed with a speckled veil which could not hide the sly charm of her face.... [She] drew closer. It was she, the creature forever yearned for ...; the time for the train's departure must be very close. When she was face-to-face with him she raised her veil, and there, chaste but ready for possession, she looked lovelier than she ever had when glimpsed in stellar space."

◆◆◆

Perhaps we should talk less about death and more about dying. And not be afraid of the subject, not push it away. "It is a matter of prime importance for the ordinary man who, by contrast with the doctor, may only encounter death once, or maybe a few times in his entire life." And then he has to cope alone—for better or worse—when it happens to him. Because: "But a common night awaiteth every man, and Death's path must be trodden once for all."

Various paths lead us to death. Incurable progressive illnesses are often the starting point for one of them, illnesses that keep marching forward relentlessly, destroying and laying waste until they have exhausted all possible forms of treatment. Then palliative medicine comes to the patient's aid, caring for him at the close of life. Its name comes from the Latin words *palliare*, meaning "to wrap or cover," and *pallium*, meaning "an overcoat," and so it involves "wrapping an overcoat" around abandoned patients whom medicine designed to find a cure can no longer help. We associate palliative and hospice medicine with soothing pain and with sedation, in other words, applying drugs that dull awareness for patients who are suffering greatly. Indeed, that is a feature of its effect, but by no means the only one, because it is performed by a qualified team of caregivers (doctor, nurse, social worker, psychologist, chaplain, physiotherapist, volunteer) and should be available, first and foremost, as a round-the-clock home counseling service or at a day-care center, or ultimately a full-time nursing home. It is estimated that of the nearly four hundred thousand people dying of chronic illnesses in Poland each year (including about a hundred thousand who die of malignant tumors), more than half require palliative care.

We would all hope to be sure of a dignified death, without suffering, and to benefit from the loving presence of someone dear to us, and some solid support and reliable information about terminal illness, "essential for closing the most important stage—the end of life." Meanwhile, the carers avoid tricky questions by fobbing the dying person off with perfunctory answers. Many families do so in league, feeding them false hopes for a chance of getting better, and denying the inevitable approach of death. And how many of us doctors are incapable of talking to dying patients, avoid contact with them and limit ourselves simply to prescribing drugs, often without discussions with the family. Eventually, the moment comes when it is too late for that deferred, neglected contact. This is the agony of death — just over two-thirds of patients partially or entirely lose consciousness in the final twenty-four hours of life.

A person who is incurably sick, especially as he approaches death, does not just suffer physically but also spiritually, existentially. His sense of isolation increases — "the metaphysical isolation of a man who is passing over into death, the great chasm of the unknown," a feeling so strong that even true believers think God has abandoned them at such a moment. Questions about the meaning of human existence keep insistently recurring, prompted by suffering and the fear that comes with it, rather than by a theoretical interest in philosophy. A troubled conscience increases the dying person's sense of responsibility for life, for the wrong he has done. How important it is to be at his side just then! However, we do not need to fill these moments with advice and consolation. We do need to listen. "One should not fear silence." Or drown out the dying person's thoughts. Sometimes it is hard to find the answers to his questions, and he is aware that we do not know them. But we do not need to be in a hurry to explain, or feel ashamed of our helplessness. Usually the best answer to those questions is our loving, devoted presence.

Can we possibly fail to think of the Polish Pope in this context? John Paul II always did his best to visit the sick and to be with people who were suffering, and he thought about suffering very thoroughly. But then a time came, the final stage, when he could no longer write or speak about suffering, and instead he became suffering. And then through his own example he showed us how, by strength of spirit and faith, it is possible to overcome suffering and, by one's own suffering, enrich the lives of millions—something that had seemed impossible, because a time comes when the suffering goes beyond measure, when the bond breaks and the sick person is shut away from us in some other world.

But he knew that this bond with us—made of the same fabric as the bond with heaven that we are always breaking—should never be broken. And when we saw him for the last time, on Easter Sunday at a window of the Apostolic Palace, he was still trying to share his words with us, even though he could not. Perhaps he was hoping to cheer us up, as he had done so many times in the past? Or maybe, as on the final page he wrote on his deathbed with the help of his entourage, he wanted to thank the young people whom he had sought out all his life and who had now come from all over the world to be with him? We will never know what else he wanted to say, but he left us the image of himself at the window, when the words could no longer come out, but he raised his drooping arms, as if trying to embrace us, as if he were saying goodbye with them, like the wings of a mortally wounded bird as it flies away ...

He also showed us how it is possible to die, and how a person should die. He invited us to keep him company in death. Some people thought it rather a pitiless novelty, admitted one eminent writer who is an avowed atheist, to show that "one does not die in isolation or seclusion, but in the public gaze; but then that is exactly how Jesus died." He showed that a person who is completely immobilized, nailed to a cross, unable to utter any words, can do a great deal. He showed this to a world that wants to be young forever and has pushed dying and death out of its conscious mind, denying them the right to exist. Are we not often like the people in Brueghel's painting *The Fall of Icarus* who cannot even be distracted from their mindless, everyday occupations by something as astonishing as a boy falling from the sky right next to them? Everyone calmly walks away from misfortune.

Death kept pace with John Paul II throughout his life, from the loss of his mother in childhood, and soon after his father too, through to the assassination attempt of May 1981. During his pontificate he was in the hospital twelve times in the Gemelli clinic and had numerous operations. In his final years his illness advanced, and we watched with aching hearts as he looked ill and visibly suffered. Yet at the same time, to the very end his suffering went hand in hand with courage, great persistence and determination. He even accepted his increasing lack of mobility with good humor, jokingly calling his mobile platform a "wheelbarrow." "Anyone who witnessed the passing of John Paul II will remain cautious in presenting some of the arguments about euthanasia."

The Pope taught us that we should accept pain and suffering fully and totally, and no one could possibly have sounded more convincing when he said that a vocation for suffering is a way of sharing in the suffering of Christ. He showed us the mysteries of suffering and death. Without him we were ready to forget they exist. We did not know how to take them on board, but we did know that he understood them and could introduce them to us — with his entire self, his teaching, his life and death.

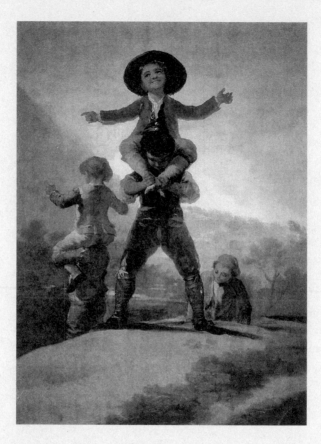

Francisco Goya
Game of the Little Giants, 1792–1793
Prado, Madrid

PROMETHEAN AMBITIONS

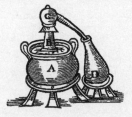

In 1955 President Dwight D. Eisenhower had a heart attack. He was given morphine, put to bed and told to stay there for four weeks. In a heart attack, or myocardial infarction, the sudden closure of the coronary artery leads to the demise of the part of the cardiac muscle that was nourished by this artery. Thus it was believed that lying flat for a month facilitates healing within the damaged heart and helps produce a strong, tight scar. Forty-five years later, U.S. vice president Dick Cheney suffered an infarction: at the hospital a coronary catheterization was immediately performed, and the closed branch of the artery was identified and opened by introducing a small balloon. The patient was given strong anticoagulant drugs, and after four days he left the hospital in good form, on his own two legs. What a fundamental difference in treatment methods!

Coronary artery angioplasty, as the opening of a closed artery is called, usually supported by implanting a stent, in other words, a delicate metal scaffold that keeps the blood vessel open, helps the patient to survive the toughest stage of the illness and often saves his life. If it is performed early, in the first few hours of sickness, it reduces the area of the infarction. But even so, part of the muscle dies for good, especially as many patients don't reach the hospital quickly. If only it were possible to revive that dying area! If only we could introduce new cells in that spot, that would take over the function of the ones destroyed by the infarction. Such an idea could have wide application in treatment, leading to the medical break-through of the twenty-first century. Indeed, infarctions develop not just in the heart but also in the brain, lungs and many other organs. In each case tens, hundreds of thousands of cells die. Just as much, or sometimes even more, damage occurs without an infarc-tion, for example when the spine is broken and the spinal cord is injured, or in diseases such as Parkinson's, Alzheimer's and other degenerative brain conditions. In all of them, regeneration of the damaged areas could reverse the course of the illness. The dream solution would be young, developing cells full of energy, which when injected into the disease-affected organ would transform into its own cells and restore its healthy functioning. You have probably guessed, Reader, that our sights are set on stem cells. It is on them, above all, that medicine is placing its great hopes.

So what are these creatures on which we are pinning so much hope? They are the primary cells from which specialized cells develop. It is from them that the cells of the muscles, liver, bones and brain originate. They are the stem from which the branches of the tree grow; this central feature has given them their name. But the root of their Polish name, *komórki macierzyste*, which means literally "maternal cells," is apt too, because it refers to the mother who gives birth to offspring.

Where can we find them? How can we obtain them? They lie dormant in most of our tissues and organs, but they are scattered and not numerous. There are a few more of them, though still not many, in the blood. However, their main storehouse is the bone marrow. It is there that the remaining blood cells develop from them — red, white, and all the others. From the bone marrow, the stem cells make their way into the blood system and probably settle in at least some of the organs.

Cells gathered from the bone marrow were first injected into patients in an area of the heart altered by an infarction at the start of the current century. The first reports were electrifying. They spoke of a rise in the contractibility of the heart muscle of as much as thirty percent. But in the latest, comprehensive publications a note of skepticism has already emerged. We should remember, however, that the groups treated so far are still very few in number. A transplant of cells is usually combined with revascularization, or an improvement in the blood supply by means of a simultaneous angioplasty and stent implant. Thus it can be quite impossible to determine what has produced the favorable result of these operations. We discovered for ourselves how hard it is to assess this promising course of action when, after reading the first article published by Japanese scientists on treating atherosclerosis of the arteries of the lower limbs, we conducted similar experiments at our hospital. So far they have included only about a dozen people with advanced lower limb ischemia in the course of Buerger's disease or atherosclerosis. These were patients with constant pain at rest and non-healing ulcers or superficial necrosis of the feet, which were already under threat of amputation. We collected bone marrow from each patient's ilium, and after brief preparation we injected it subcutaneously into the muscles of the foot or calf in at least forty places. The first striking effect was a cessation of pain one or two days later, enabling a radical reduction of analgesics. In over half the patients the necrosis gradually lessened and the healing process for the ulcers began, which was confirmed by angiographic tests that indicated an expansion of the network of vessels of the shin and foot and an increase in the blood flow. But in some patients the illness progressed, resulting in amputation. So are there patients who react to this treatment, and others whom it leaves unaffected? How can we tell them apart? And how much auto-suggestion is there in all this for a patient who is already expecting amputation and who is suddenly offered hope? The cold observer will say the group we treated was too small to draw any binding conclusions, and he will be right. He will also add that it is essential to conduct the experiments using a placebo, so that half the patients are injected with physiological saline instead of bone marrow, and neither doctor nor patient will know who has been given what until the end of the experiment, when the code disguising the patients' names is revealed. Without doing this, the cold observer will say, you will never know the truth. And he will be right. But if we keep hearing the happy chirping of cardiologists all around us, announcing fabulous results in infarction cases, what is to stop us from applying the same treatment to patients with chronic lower limb ischemia? Or to those who have already been through every degree of suffering? Are we to inject physiological saline into painful areas and keep an eye on them for over a month? But without doing that, won't we keep wandering in the dark forever? It is extremely likely, and our results will certainly never be regarded as credible. After the initial, open attempt at treatment, randomized research involving a double blind test will be essential. This example illustrates the modern requirements for new forms of therapy.

I shall cite an unusual example of the application of stem cells. A young Catalan woman, the mother of two children, fell ill in 2004 with tuberculosis. The illness took a severe course and refused to respond to drugs. The tubercular swellings were blocking her airway. In 2007 the diameter of the trachea contracted to four millimeters. The trachea was removed, a fusion with the bronchus was made and a stent was put in, but none of this helped, and the patient continued to suffocate day and night. Then something unusual was done. Stem cells were taken from the patient's bone marrow, as well as cells from her airway, and these were sent to a laboratory in Bristol, England, to be multiplied in vitro. At the same time, the trachea was removed from the body of a fifty-one-year-old woman who had died of a brain hemorrhage. It was totally cleansed of its own cells, and also sent to Bristol, where, in a bioreactor flown in from Milan, it was seeded with our patient's previously multiplied stem cells. These cells took root in the trachea and grew over it. And so a new trachea was produced, the solid structure of which, the skeleton, came from a dead patient, but the walls of which were made from cells taken from the living patient waiting for a transplant. Meanwhile, time was rushing by, and the patient's condition worsened abruptly. A regular flight from Bristol to Barcelona refused to take the "manufactured" trachea on board, but fortunately a German student on his practical training tracked down a friend with a private plane, who flew to Barcelona in time. The colonized windpipe was implanted into our patient, and as the cells were the patient's own, the transplant took perfectly, with no rejection — the bane of this sort of procedure. Apparently, three months later the patient, a fiery thirty-year-old woman, danced half the night away at a ball on the Costa Brava.

The substance we implant from the bone marrow is composite material. Here too some people perceive divergent results for treating heart attacks, and they say: "Mixed cells give mixed results." If only we had pure stem cells! But of course we do have them — they appear in fetal life, at the very start, before the diversification stage. It is from them, these primal embryonic stem cells, that the cells of the heart, liver, brain and other organs will later develop. Human embryonic stem cells could be obtained by means of cloning. What does cloning involve? The nucleus is removed from an egg cell and another nucleus is put in its place, taken from the cell of a mature organism. Then an incredible, mysterious reaction occurs: the nucleus radically rejuvenates; the hands on the clock go back to the beginning, to the embryonic state. In this mature nucleus, under the influence of "female" cytoplasm, genes are aroused that were active a long time ago, in fetal life, but were then extinguished. The cloned egg cells, with their mysteriously reprogrammed nuclei, are implanted into the uterus of an adoptive mother, and months later she bears a child. So in 1997 Dolly the lamb was cloned, and after her other sheep, cows, a horse, a piglet, a wolf, a mouflon, a buffalo, a donkey, a mule, a cat, a dog ... Ten years after Dolly's birth her creator, Ian Wilmut, says: "we should still be surprised that cloning works at all." Another renowned biotechnologist agrees with him, asserting: "cloning is still essentially a black box" — its workings are incomprehensible. Its efficiency is also far below expectations. Nowadays, only from two to four percent of cloned animal embryos are born as healthy individuals. That is not much better than ten years ago. Of two hundred and seventy-seven cloned embryos, Dolly was the only one to be born and to have survived.

Reproductive cloning, in other words, experiments aimed at reproducing a complete human being, is against the law in all countries. But for using stem cells for scientific research and ultimate medical purposes, the situation is different. And so there are three sources of stem cells. The first is the bone marrow, though there they are found in a highly dispersed state. The second is cloning. Here the problem is with the eggs. It is difficult for scientists to acquire enough female ova for their needs, and so they pay volunteers enormous sums of money for them. The third source is human embryos from the period before they take root in the uterus (blastocytes), which are available at clinics treating infertility (with in vitro fertilization), where they are sometimes obtained in excess, as so-called surplus embryos. They are doomed to perish, or to be preserved in a frozen state, if the parents envisage further pregnancies. Both cloning and the manipulation of early-stage human embryos prompt serious ethical objections and are the subject of a wide range of regulations in different countries.

All these difficulties and obstacles may be mitigated by a new approach, involving a revolutionary concept. What if, the thinking goes, one were to reprogram a mature, developed somatic cell without the help of the cytoplasm of an egg cell? What if one were to work directly on its DNA, and wake up the genes that are dormant within it and have been inactive since the embryo stage? This fantastic vision became a reality at the turn of 2007 and 2008, thanks to Japanese scientist Shinya Yamanaka. He took mature cells (from the facial skin of a grown woman) and introduced into them four genes (in specialized terms known as "transcription factors"). A month later, they had transformed the cells into human stem cells (in specialized terms "induced, Pluripotent Stem Cells," or iPSCs). Thus a mature cell had reverted many years backwards, to the earliest stage of its existence, to begin life over again so to speak. These results have already been confirmed in many laboratories. Yamanaka, a forty-nine-year-old scientist from Kyoto who had wanted to be an orthopedist but took up research when he realized he did not have the manual skills, recently won the Lasker Award, which is the last step before the Nobel Prize.

But there is no doubt that a breakthrough has been made, a shake-up in the scientific world. Ian Wilmut, creator of Dolly the sheep, said that from now on he would stop experimenting on human embryonic stem cells, because the new discoveries opened up far more interesting prospects. And something just as important: they have eliminated a weighty ethical problem. To recreate stem cells in the future, it will not be necessary to turn to human reproductive cells or embryos. Those whose lives are consumed by cloning but made unpleasant by ethics are also aware of this. On first hearing about the breakthrough discovery described here, one of them announced with satisfaction: "People working on ethics will have to find something new to worry about!"

With the help of this particular method — the reprogramming of mature cells — stem cells have already been obtained from patients with Down syndrome, muscular dystrophy, insulin-dependent diabetes and dozens of other hereditary illnesses. These cells are multiplied in a culture, and are long-lived. The plan is to remove from them the defective genes responsible for the illness, implant normal genes, and inject the patients with these "repaired" stem cells — and thus to correct a defective mutation permanently. Stem cells obtained from patients can also be transformed into the more mature cells of individual organs (e.g., the cells of the heart muscle) in order to test their response to drugs.

However, the road to clinical application is immeasurably long and abounding in difficulties. The vehicle that introduced the four reprogrammed genes into the mature cells (the "transcription factors") are viruses that also carry countless dangers, including the potential to cause cancer. Similarly, in the stem cells themselves the potential to cause cancer is strong. The first doubts are also appearing as to whether during the reprogramming process "genetic and epigenetic abnormalities in the iPSCs" might result, which would call into question their future application in medical treatment.

There is also the issue of time. The flow of time, the relentless passage from past into future, is one of mankind's most basic experiences, a fundamental feature of reality. We talk about the arrow of time and it is an apt metaphor since, just like a flying arrow, time does not keep still, but races irreversibly in the direction the arrowhead is pointing. However, it is not always perceived like that. In music, the linear passage of time didn't take hold until in the works of Mozart, Haydn and Beethoven, marking the advent of musical modernity. We define the arrow of time as cosmological when we wish to stress the existence of one common time for the entire Universe (which is not at odds with the theory of relativity, according to which the passage of time is different within different frames of reference). For indeed the Universe is expanding, galaxies are moving apart, and as this process continues the density of matter diminishes, and of two states of the Universe, the one where the density of matter is now greater is the earlier.

By reprogramming a cell we reset its time to the earliest stages of its life. It does not seem right to say that we have turned back the arrow of time. After all, time has not run in the opposite direction; it wasn't that a movie has been run backwards from a certain point, or a tape gradually rewound. Instead, intuition tells us that time, like the hands on a clock face, has turned a circle and gone back to its beginning. The words of Pythagoras come to mind: "the world turns a circle," and so does the Greek Stoics' idea of eternal return and the cyclical nature of the world's history. After each cycle the world was meant to return to its primordial state (*apokatastasis*) and exactly the same structure was rebuilt. Nietzsche was particularly fond of this concept, which re-echoes nowadays in Henri Poincaré's famous recurrence theorem, and also in Kurt Gödel's closed timelike curves, which set off a landslide of works about time loops.

The large number of legal regulations, their diversity and spread between extremes, reflect the temperature of ongoing debate around the world concerning the ethical grounds for cloning and interfering with the origins of life. The truly phenomenal development of the sciences, especially biology, seems to be prompting questions that were quite unknown to previous generations. Yet they are echoes of the questions and tests that have been with us since almost the dawn of history. How did man come to be?

Could man alone, by his own art, produce living creatures, or even another human being? And is it at all possible to produce life from inanimate matter? Yes, was the reply to that question given in the sixth century BC by Anaximander of Miletus, who stated that sea creatures arise straight from earth and water under the hot rays of the sun. Therefore man could have come into the world from fish, having been born in the form of a shark. This theory was deduced from observations of natural phenomena: a certain species of shark (*Mustelus laevis*) gives birth to its young and does not lay eggs. So the idea of life spontaneously appearing had already surfaced several hundred years before Aristotle supported and developed it in his treatises. For hundreds of years people believed that from one species of declining fauna another could arise. In his *Metamorphoses* Ovid describes how bees emerged out of the decaying bodies of cows, wasps out of horses and scorpions out of crab shells, and in the fourth book of Virgil's *Georgics* there is a recipe for making bees hatch out of a dying bull calf. And indeed, more than fifteen hundred years later John Locke—the founder of empiricist philosophy, the major scholarly trend of the Enlightenment—a man of moderate and sober mind, in his manuscript "To Make a Toad or Serpent," gave a detailed description, rich in technical minutiae, of the enterprise defined in the title that begins with boiling a goose or duck over a slow fire. It ends with the assurance that a certain doctor from Poland, using the given recipe, produced works of creation as many as six times, to which the Duke of Hannover can testify, having watched him in wonder and amazement.

We too, following the Duke of Hannover's example, are filled with admiration for the skills of our colleague and compatriot. But what is the use, we may ask, of yet another toad or yet another serpent? To create a man would be the summit of arcane knowledge! The first news of it comes from third-century Egypt. It is the story of Salaman and Absala. It takes us back to ancient times, when King Harmanus ruled the kingdom of Rum, which covered Egypt, the shores of the Mediterranean Sea and Greece. The king is childless, but at the thought of intimacy with a woman he is overcome by a strange disgust. So for help and advice he turns to his divine counselor Qualiqulas, an ascetic who has already lived for thirty generations, dividing his time between educating the king in the sciences and solitary contemplation in the cave of Serapeion, aiming his thoughts towards perfection and a life of purity. After some hesitation the king agrees to the master's suggestion to conceive an heir by artificial means. Qualiqulas puts the king's semen in a bottle the shape of a mandragora and by his mysterious art causes a human being to appear, equipped with a soul. Salaman, for that is the name given to the boy, is suckled by a beautiful young girl named Absala. When he grows up, he falls madly in love with her and she with him, but the king soon becomes an obstruction, expecting his one and only son and heir to turn his mind and soul towards the world of ideals. The lovers run away from the king. Ever-greater obstacles pile up in front of them, until finally, to remain together forever, they decide on a suicide pact. She drowns, but he is saved at the last moment by a sea spirit. Insane with longing, he dreams of just one thing—to see her once again. So Qualiqulas summons up the spirit of Absala, having first obtained the young man's pledge that he will spend forty days alone with him, meditating in the cave of Serapeion. What death has failed to do, Aphrodite almost achieves, by appearing more and more often to Salaman instead of Absala. But finally he rejects carnal temptations and, in accordance with his father's wishes, takes over the kingdom.

This tale was listened to for centuries, and even the Persian sage and great doctor Avicenna wrote about it. In modern times the cave has even been located where Qualiqulas is meant to have devoted himself to his meditations. It has also been noted that the names of the heroes may have their origins in the remote past in Sanskrit: Salaman may have been derived from *Sraman*, meaning "ascetic," and Absala from *Absara*, a succubus sent to tempt ascetics. Regardless of its Platonic elements, this story tells us for the first time of the artificial creation of a human being from the semen of a man and is the starting point for the history of the homunculus, which will carry on for centuries, reaching its zenith with Paracelsus.

Bathed in glory, the miracle-working doctor Paracelsus was a restless, adventurous soul. Ever on the move, he traveled about on horseback, practiced in different countries with consistent staggering success, wrote by night and slept with a sword at his side. From a portrait of him by Rubens in the Musée Royal des Beaux Arts in Brussels, his piercing gaze stares out at us from under flame-red hair. He has a solid build and his face is rather puffy, because he did not deny himself alcohol. His remains, preserved in the church of Saint Sebastian in Salzburg, where he died in 1541, have undergone detailed analysis. From the measurement of his pelvis and long bones, there has even been an attempt to draw the conclusion that his gender could just as well have been female as male! He proclaimed that medicine should preoccupy the whole doctor, as his subject was the whole human body. Though in the pommel of the sword from which he was never parted he had a hollow sphere full of pills for his patients, in his writings he repeated that "the best medicine is love." He went his own way, and encouraged others to do so to the maximum: "Let no man belong to another that can belong to himself" (*Alterius non sit, qui suus esse potest*).

Paracelsus and his predecessors and imitators created the image of the alchemist as a *magus coelestis*, a sorcerer close to divine creative powers. In working together to refine matter, they aimed at their own perfection. While, a few hundred years earlier, alchemy had already been a powerful magnet for restless, inquiring minds, it was only Paracelsus and his contemporaries who pushed it to the limits of its potential. Its crowning achievement was the homunculus, the artificial man, affording his creator the position of a quasi-demiurge, a virtual god. It was the ultimate act in man's domination of nature, the mystery of all mysteries. It was produced from a man's semen, kept warm for forty days. Towards the end of this period the ethereal outline of a transparent, incorporeal man emerged. After another forty days, fed sporadically on blood, it took on a human shape as if born from a woman, but smaller. In its mature form it possessed might and rare abilities, because it was a work of art. It did not need to learn from others; it came knowing mysteries and arcane matters.

Goethe knew the recipe for creating a homunculus from a book ascribed to Paracelsus called *De natura rerum* and made certain changes to it. In the second book of *Faust*, Wagner, the Master's pedantic assistant, toils away in the fairytale alchemist's laboratory, unsuccessfully trying to create a man in a retort. He explains to Mephistopheles, who is watching him, that he has mixed hundreds of substances and subjected them to repeated distillation, in the hope that the expected, live result will finally crystallize. It is only Mephistopheles's magical power that brings the enterprise to a successful end. Out of the chaos of unformed matter a tiny, well-shaped little man emerges who instantly engages in a philosophical dispute, inspired by being shut in the glass confines around him. The homunculus, Faust and Mephistopheles leave Wagner with his fat alchemy books and set off for Thessaly on Walpurgis night. There the homunculus launches a lively debate with Thales and Anaxagoras. Proteus joins them, and advises him that to achieve mature existence he should travel with him to the high seas. Only in the boundless expanse of the waters will he be free "to move in all dimensions and directions." Stunned by the beauty of the ocean and the strength of the emotion arising within him, the homunculus smashes the glass bottle keeping him captive. And then, in a flash of light, the little figure evaporates forever. In a conversation with Eckermann, Goethe stressed the superiority of the homunculus over Mephistopheles because of his "tendency to the beautiful, and to a useful activity." He has been compared to Plato's daimon, though, of course, he was derived from Paracelsus's tradition as an incorporeal creature that knows the secrets of arcane matters. For Goethe he was "a symbol for the human intellect and its liberating capabilities."

But in Judaism things were different. Jewish thought produced one of the most intriguing ideas — the golem. It prefigured Adam, and an early stage in the effort to create it appears in the Talmud. However, only from the thirteenth century, among the Ashkenazi Hasidim, does the golem start to signify an artificial man. When the rabbi set about creating a golem, first of all he fasted for five days, then he molded the little figure of a man from mud and clay and said to it: *Shem ha-meforash*, meaning "the distinguished Name of God," and on its forehead he wrote: *emet*, meaning "truth." This word contains the Hebrew alphabet, from *aleph* to *tav*. Written in a mystic trance, among linguistic permutations, it achieved its aim: the little figure came to life. Although it could not speak, it understood what was said to it, and did all the housework, although it was not allowed to leave the Jewish home. It grew slowly, but steadily, turning into the golem, who surpassed the household in strength and height. Once it became a threat to them, the first letter was wiped from its brow, and *emet* was transformed into *met*, which means "dead." Then the golem disintegrated into the bits of clay from which it had arisen. According to legend, the golem created by the tzaddik Elias Baal Shem of Chełm grew to such a height that the tzaddik could no longer reach his brow. So he told the giant to bow down and take off his boots, so he could change the inscription on its forehead. And so it happened. But as the golem collapsed into lumps of clay and mud, it buried him and crushed him, like the sorcerer's apprentice.

The most famous golem was created in the sixteenth century in Prague by the alchemist, kabbalist and astronomer to the Emperor Rudolph II, Rabbi Judah Loew ben Bezalel, to defend the persecuted Jewish community. Thanks to its superhuman strength, the golem performed its duties excellently. But one day it went berserk and started blindly sowing destruction, and the decision was made to destroy it. Echoes of this story resound in the novel *Frankenstein, or the Modern Prometheus* by Mary Shelley, second wife of the poet Percy Bysshe Shelley. The novel was written in Switzerland, where the Shelleys and Byron spent a rainy summer amusing themselves by writing ghost stories. In her story Frankenstein, the Genevan philosophy student, discovers the secret of animating matter. Using body parts stolen from graveyards and mortuaries, he creates the repulsive, powerful monster, who feels lonely and unhappy. In vengeance against his creator, he commits some dreadful crimes and finally takes his own life. In popular culture through the years, especially under the influence of the movie versions, the name "Frankenstein" came to stand for the monster himself, and not his creator, the modern Prometheus.

The successive incarnations of the golem and Frankenstein inspired terror with their superhuman size and insuperable strength. Terror overcame the gods on Olympus for the first time when the giants, offspring of Gaia, the Earth, born from the blood that ran from the wounds of her husband, Ouranos, came into the world.

As soon as they were born they threatened the heavens, hurling up burning trees and mighty rocks. The gigantomachia was the toughest war the gods ever fought, and the horror of these battles is shown to us on the pediments of Greek temples. Dante encountered the defeated giants in hell. Their torsos and huge hands petrified him and filled him with fear, and so he said with relief:

> Nature did well to leave off making these
> Creatures and other creatures like them, taking
> Such monstrous ministers away from Mars.
> And, though she still continues with the whale
> And elephant, if one considers subtly,
> That turns out to be well advised as well.

As I write this, I remember my own particular experience in this respect. Once, when I was a young doctor in Wrocław, I was just starting one of my first shifts. On a sunny afternoon I was walking down a long, bright hospital corridor under the high vaults of neo-Gothic arches. Ahead of me there was a bend curving at a right-angle, and then just a straight stretch to the ward. Suddenly from around the bend in the corridor a shadow loomed towards me. It grew, and quick as blinking it had filled the whole space with darkness. I felt a chill and a rush of inexplicable fear. The idea of a solar eclipse had just crossed my mind when from around the bend a giant emerged. He was bearing down on me, filling the entire corridor. As we passed each other, I shrank against the wall and heard a voice booming somewhere high above my head: "Good evening, Doctor." I sighed with relief. That was my first encounter with Michasio, our giant, an acromegalic.

In the rare illness of gigantism, in childhood or very early youth the pituitary gland produces an excess of growth hormone, and the person grows and grows until he reaches superhuman proportions.

The tallest giant recorded in medical chronicles was eight feet, seven inches high. Our Michasio was eight feet, three inches. We invited him to the hospital two or three times a year, not just for treatment, but also to show him to the students. Special preparations were made in advance of his admission, because we had nothing for him to lie on. I well remember how a nurse and I dismantled a hospital bed, attached a table to its legs, and then another smaller table, and then covered it all in mattresses. Michasio's fellow patients on the ward, their masculinity fired, often wanted to arm-wrestle with him. Without any enthusiasm he would accept these challenges, and in a couple of seconds settle them to his advantage.

By nature he was gentle and cheerful, and did not flaunt his strength. He liked to arrange flowers, embroider and play chess. He found the perfect job, at Jelcz, a car factory in a Wrocław suburb, where he painted the buses. As he used to take pleasure in saying: "With me there, they don't need a ladder."

The giant, whom a doctor will meet at best once or twice in his professional career, provides a reminder of the mythical origins of the world. He also reminds us of the times when people tried to create an artificial man. There was one question that bothered all these creators — alchemists, magicians, shamans or doctors. It was not a technical one, or anything to do with the recipe. It was this: Do they have a soul? Making the magic come true, realizing it to perfection depended on the answer, because if the little men out of a retort, the homunculi and golems, were not meant to have souls, what exactly were they? Sub-humans? Surrogates? Soulless robots? In the story of Salaman and Absala, we read that the homunculus who arose from the king's semen, transformed inside a bottle shaped like a mandragora, was given a "rational soul." We are not surprised, as we are dealing with a moral tale that aims to describe the passage of the soul from the world of matter into the reality of ideal, universal forms. Questions about the soul worried people in the Middle Ages too. For centuries a tale was told about a famous Catalan doctor, Arnaldo of Villanova, who at the last moment was overcome by fear of mortal sin and smashed the retort containing maturing semen when the shapes of a homunculus's body started to emerge from it. The Catholic theologians had to speak out against the popular spread of attempts at artificially creating people. Reviling the charlatans and citing reasons why the enterprise was impossible, they sometimes resorted to some astonishing logic. Thus one of these seventeenth-century arguments stated that the soul of a homunculus, created *de novo*, would be devoid of the original sin passed down to us from Adam, and so the homunculus would not need salvation through Christ. Proof indeed via a *reductio ad absurdum*.

Meanwhile, Judaism found an ingenious way to solve the problem of the soul by introducing gradations for it. The transformation of inanimate chaos into a well-shaped being, into a golem, ends with giving him the lowest soul (the *nefesh*) by branding his face with the word *emet*. In the hierarchy, the golem's soul (the *nefesh*) is inferior to the higher soul of Adam (the *neshama*). A being produced by the hand of man is not equal in perfection to the work of the Creator.

Increasingly often, we read that cloning human beings is an inevitable business, and we could start to believe the process is near to happening. Science fiction features discussions on the souls of clones. The story of the rise and fall of Hwang Woo-suk, mentioned earlier, should stand as a warning to us. In 2004–2005 this renowned Korean scientist, who had cloned an Afghan hound before then, published several papers in prestigious journals on procuring the first human embryonic stem cells, showing pictures of them. The way forwards for regenerative medicine lay open. We were to regain our lost capacity for perfect regeneration, as preserved by the salamander, the newt or the hydra. And cloning an entire human being was inevitably approaching. The Korean team was the talk of the whole world, which for several years now had placed its greatest hopes in this field. In California, to bypass the ethical provisos of the federal government, three billion dollars were allocated from the state budget and work was begun to create a cloning center. Other states followed this example. At the height of these expectations it was discovered that Hwang's results were a fraud, one of the biggest in the modern history of science. In just a few weeks Hwang, the national hero, admired by the world, lost everything, including his honor and university post. The flagship Korean airlines took away the free lifelong first-class air ticket they had awarded him earlier. The postage stamps depicting a wheelchair-bound patient leaping to his feet after an injection of stem cells were withdrawn from circulation. For a while the whole field, regarded as the most important in biology and as the future of medicine, was under a dark cloud.

The icon of regenerative medicine should really be Prometheus, whose liver was eaten by a vulture on a daily basis for thirty thousand years but grew back each night. The liver's ability to regenerate is confirmed by modern medicine, which contrasts that organ with the heart muscle. The popular myth of Prometheus has various original versions, because myths were nomadic tales, and the Greeks were accustomed to the idea that the same stories could be heard in different versions. And so, by being flexible, the myth avoided becoming ritual. It was a story that was composed over and over again, each time becoming slightly different. Something might be left out, and something else added. These variants "keep the mythical blood in circulation." Thanks to this, the myth could "breathe deeper" within literature.

According to one version, man was created by Prometheus, who molded him out of clay mixed with tears. In Boeotia until recently there was a hut on display where Prometheus did his work. Around it lay lumps of clay-like red earth emitting an odor that smelled like a human body. The first people wandered about "like faint apparitions out of dreams," helpless against the might of nature. Then Prometheus crept into heaven, stole a spark and carried it down for the mortals. Fire gave people power over all creatures on Earth, because it was part of the power of the gods. For this deed Zeus stunned Prometheus with a thunderbolt and chained him to a cliff in the Caucasus, where the vulture daily ate his liver until Heracles released him from this torment.

The myth of Prometheus, one of the noblest characters in mythology, had a very strong power to influence and has been expressed in art like few others. Aeschylus's tragedy *Prometheus Bound* had already shaped him for rebellion against tyranny and a relentless fight for the happiness of mankind and freedom of spirit, ending, after immeasurable sufferings, in victory. And so it went for centuries: in the poetry of Goethe, Mickiewicz and Shelley, in Beethoven's overtures, symphonic poems by Liszt and Skriabin, and paintings by Titian and Rubens. Promethean fire would forever be associated with the spark of the gods, inspiration, heroic courage and creative force. All those who have tried or try to create man *de novo*, outside the forces of nature — as a homunculus, golem or clone — they all have their origin in Prometheus. They have turned to magic, the *Ars Magna* and its reflections in

Judaism—the alchemy of the word—and finally, in modern times, to molecular biology, in order to know just a fraction of the mystery that belongs in its entirety to God alone.

Shackled to the rock, in a conversation with Zeus, Prometheus says that he brought man freedom by giving him fire. He broke the chains that made him a prisoner of the gods' laws, and set him free to achieve humanity, to create himself. To which Zeus just as splendidly replies:

> *You think you freed him? You separated him*
> *From the illumination of heaven,*
> *From the wisdom and certainty of heaven.*
> *You freed him*
> *To grope his way into the mine shaft, into the bank vault*
> *Of his own ego, his selfishness*
> *And his pride. . . .*
> *You cut the nerves*
> *That connected him to his own soul. . . .*
> *When man has learned to live without his soul*
> *I shall be redundant . . .*
> *His ears will fill up with different voices . . .*

These words imply a profound lack in the human condition, a hidden contradiction. That is why man appears torn "between good and evil, strength and weakness, wisdom and the desires that control him, between what is small and what is great, lust and virtual sainthood, truth and appearance." His tragic fate makes it impossible for him to be an unambiguous figure. And man stands facing a border that pride tells him to cross. He is ready to use force or violence to get beyond this border.

◆◆◆

The great Greek tragedians knew all about *hybris* and *hamartia*, unrestrained pride, the ambition to cast off the fetters of prohibitive rules and norms, to gain absolute freedom at any price. Nowadays only the scenery has changed, while our nature has remained the same. However, for a doctor it is harder to find a foothold in the modern world, where postmodernism promotes "a model of life that is not conditioned by norms," a limitless pluralism of beliefs, relativism, a mild global outlook and uncritical consent for all manner of strange and alternative behavior; a world that is animated by the will to demystify authority and to deconstruct, and that also brushes aside the question about the meaning of existence, a meaning that is established without our involvement and perceived in an act of amazement. Where should we seek the limits of freedom? These questions are especially close to medicine, whose patron, Asclepius, went beyond the limits of the human sphere of existence by resurrecting the dead, for which he was struck down by a thunderbolt. So how are we to delineate the border beyond which biotechnology should not interfere in our organism? What, after all, are we trying to protect it from? The essence of our humanity, the kernel in which man's dignity lies and the laws resulting from it? The concept of man's dignity, as the leading theme of John Paul II's pontificate, now stands before us with astonishing relevance. The border Asclepius crossed does exist, even though it is so hard for our eyes to see it.

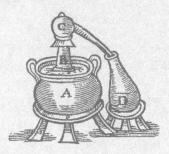

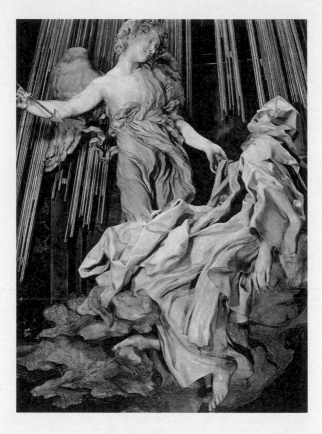

Giovanni Lorenzo Bernini
Ecstasy of Saint Teresa, 1645–1652
Cornaro Chapel, Santa Maria della Vittoria, Rome

THE ENCHANTMENT OF LOVE

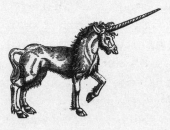

There is one illness for which the cure has been sought for centuries but never found. It is called love. There is no point in asking a doctor exactly what it is, nor will you find a description of the processes that control it in any learned medical tome. Pick up a volume of poetry instead and you will not be disappointed. You will have no trouble finding it in the theater, in a novel and in painting too — in short, in art, because it has to do with beauty. No one understood that better than Sappho:

> *Some say that the most beautiful thing on this dark earth*
> *Is a squadron of cavalry; others say*
> *A troop of infantry, others a fleet of ships;*
> *But I say that it is the one you love.*

So what has medicine got to do with love? Of course, Cupid's arrows strike doctors too, but no more often and no differently than they do other people. But maybe medicine has developed some special tool, a specialty to treat love? We may well ask such a question, if only in view of the vast number of medical specializations, which will soon be in the hundreds. Although no "love" specialty has yet been officially designated, doctors have in fact been summoned to people suffering from love sickness for centuries. Oribasius of Pergamon set about treating them in the fourth century AD. He wrote that people in love were characterized by insomnia and sadness, fluttering eyelids and sunken eyes. He pointed out the similarity to depression. He regarded unrequited, passionate, ardent love as something to be classified as a disease, an illness *sui generis* that the doctor should know how to diagnose and treat. He recommended wine, bathing, physical exercise, theater and music, stating at the same time that "the passion of those who are incessantly preoccupied by their love is difficult to uproot." He also offered a new way of distracting those unfortunates who are overwhelmed by the pain of love: you should frighten them. This principle was applied for centuries, though, as has been noted, this strategy is like suddenly and unexpectedly shouting "Boo!" at someone who has hiccups. After a period in the dark it returned in the seventeenth and eighteenth centuries, when it was also applied to the mentally ill. This renaissance of the strategy of frightening the patient is attributed to an incident described at the time in a popular medical treatise. A firmly restrained lunatic was being taken somewhere on a cart when he managed to break free of his bonds, and then jumped into a lake. After quite some time when he was finally fished out, everyone thought he was dead, but he soon recovered his senses, which turned out to have been restored to perfect order; he went on to enjoy a long life without ever experiencing madness again. Inspired by this anecdote, one doctor took to plunging madmen (including those mad with love) in fresh water or into the sea. As he claimed: "The patients should be submerged unexpectedly and held in the water for long enough. There is no fear for their lives." But Sappho and Ovid thought it impossible to be cured of love, and not even desirable. A legend that arose years after Sappho's death tells how, unable to bear an unrequited love any longer, she threw herself from the promontory of Leucadia — and that was the first love suicide. But we find the comparison of love to an illness much earlier. In about 1300 BC in an Egyptian love poem, "the beloved is described as the 'cure' and 'physician'" for the pain of the illness that is love, usually unrequited.

To suppress an inflamed imagination and silence the frenzy of love, people turned to symbolic therapy. Bienville writes about it in 1778 in his treatise *De la nymphomanie*. A significant title; the nymphs accompanied the Greek gods from time immemorial, to appear before our eyes in the Florentine *quattrocento*, after which they would never cease to gaze at us from fountains, fireplaces, balconies and balustrades. They were not just an excuse for some erotic impressions — that was not the only reason why their naked breasts or bellies might appear in one's field of vision, though "they were sometimes that too." The nymphs were also a reminder of the most dangerous kind of experience: obsession. Getting close to a nymph meant giving in to obsession; it was tantamount to "immersing yourself in a soft, mobile element, which might with equal likelihood prove thrilling or disastrous," as Roberto Calasso puts it. And although Bienville could not have known the additional dangers that nymphets would be to the hunters they bewitched, these "little deadly demons among the wholesome children" — as described by Nabokov in *Lolita* — he did know the threat of *la nymphomanie*. In his treatise Bienville offered as many as seventeen prescriptions for dousing the flames of love. Recipe number fifteen is striking, being a sort of alchemy against love: "Grind quicksilver tinged with cinnabar five times with two drachms of gold, then heat in ashes with vitriolic spirit; distil the whole five times and let stew for five hours on coal embers. Pulverize and administer three grams to the girl whose imagination is enflamed by chimeras." And so fire is treated with fire, in accordance with the eternal, magical principle that "like cures like" (*similia similibus curantur*). How could all those valuable solid bodies, consumed by fire, fail to triumph over a fever of the human body, over turmoil of the heart and mind!

Music has never been forgotten either. The healing properties ascribed to it in ancient times reappeared during the Renaissance and the Enlightenment. In the nineteenth century, cases of love obsession or even frenzy being cured by music were still being cited. It was explained as follows: the music pervades the body and decomposes into steady vibrations, and the person starts to react as if he himself were an instrument, being made to resonate harmoniously; he vibrates along with the music that is filling him. Right inside his body "the recomposition is enacted, the harmonic structure of consonance restoring the harmonious function of the passions."

However, love potions have always been in greater demand than cures for the madness of love. In ancient times the most famous one was made from the herbs of Thessaly. The Greeks called it a *philtron*. They knew it had a powerful effect, releasing the madness of love. It was these herbs, this potion, that the lovesick Phoenician queen Dido sought urgently, and in vain. She had founded a new city, Carthage, in Northern Africa. Several years later Aeneas stopped on her shores during his wanderings from the siege of Troy. A great love flares into life, but, yielding to the ancient virtue of *pietas*—the emotion due to one's family, fatherland and gods—he fulfills the wishes of the gods and decides, though with a torn heart and in defiance of Dido's entreaties, to abandon her. Then she runs herself through with a sword and throws herself on a great pyre, whose flames Aeneas sees from his ship on the open sea. As soon as she makes her decision, Dido realizes that her death is also an omen for the death of the city:

> *... she envisioned between*
> *the flame and smoke of the*
> *fire*
> *how Carthage silently*
> *crumbled*
> *ages before Cato's*
> *prophecy.*

In Poland the Thessalian herbs were replaced with native ones. Supposedly, the most effective was adder's tongue. Also in demand was a tiny fern with one small leaf, from the sheath-like base of which a thin germinal spike emerges, like the serpent protruding from the greenery to tempt Eve. The common folk called it "follow me," or "frenzied love." There were also other kinds of lovage, such as grass of Parnassus, which in the mountainous Podhale region, famous for its folklore, was also called "Adam's root" or "quaking grass." It was picked at night by moonlight, while singing a magic spell:

> *Tongue of adder, tongue of adder,*
> *Fearlessly I gather*
> *By the handful, even more,*
> *Make boys chase me by the score.*

In terms of history, no herb can compare with mandragora. It comes to us from the magical past, from the oldest folk beliefs. It was said to have originated in Eden, and was supposedly born in Paradise, and that most certainly before man was. Medicine widely took advantage of its narcotic properties. In a play by Niccolò Machiavelli, mandragora possesses sexual and fertilizing powers. It appears in the stories of Boccaccio and is often mentioned by Shakespeare as well as by Goethe in *Faust*. Its root has a human shape, and because like has an effect on like, its power extends over the entire human body. It belongs to the infamous *Solanaceae* family—the nightshades, just like the thorn-apple and other witches' herbs. It grows in graveyards or at the foot of the gallows; it grows from the last drops of a hanged man's semen.

Picking mandragora has always been linked with danger, because as soon as it feels itself being torn from the earth, the plant screams. This scream is so terrible and piercing that anyone who hears it dies. So it is best to resort to a method tried and tested for centuries. Once you have broken up the earth around the root, you tie a dog to it and place a bowl of food in front of him. The dog runs towards it and tears out the precious root. The blood-curdling scream resounds, and the dog falls dead. Hecate, goddess of the crossroads and darkness, patroness of witches, who causes people to go mad, happily accepts this sacrifice into her kingdom.

Mandragora is known to be a special herb containing particular properties. It can be "at once a source of joy and pain," both causing the madness of love and soothing it. Thus it brought the unknown, the unpredictable. In this it was like "the erotic act [which] is a leap in the dark, into the unknown." It gave you the gifts of oblivion, liberation from time and the capacity to identify completely with the moment. It let you take off on wings, and laid you open to love—the mark of eternity. But it also brought a pain that could not be separated from the ecstasy of love, the pain of uniting and the pain of parting. It was one great risk—from attempting to obtain it through to taking it. And for the sake of this risk it was so greatly sought.

The search for love potions continued nonstop for centuries. Some people, as if at the instigation of the popular London surgeon who said, "Why think? Why not try?," concocted whole ranges of potions and tried them out, often on themselves first. Others sought prescriptions in the great tomes of magicians and alchemists. They never doubted such a potion could exist, as shown by the most beautiful love story ever told, the tale of Tristan and Isolde. To marry the king of Cornwall, the beautiful, golden-haired Irish princess, Isolde, sails by ship in the care of the knight Tristan. They develop strong feelings for each other. She is driven to despair by his indifference, which is only feigned out of loyalty to his king. By mistake they drink a love potion meant for other purposes. What happens next occurs beyond their will and knowledge. From then on they are "blameless culprits, sinless sinners." We wish them luck with all our hearts, as they fall into the traps set for them. More than that, "we should forgive them all the lies, deceit, perjury and even crimes the ambiguous situation forced them into. We should hate all those who stood in the way of this great love." An audacious, adulterous love, let us add. Time has no power over the lovers, and this is at the heart of the fabulous charm of their destiny, the story of a perfect love "born not from life, but from love of life" — indisputable love.

In as recently as 2003 the prestigious *British Medical Journal* made an attempt to analyze the ingredients of the love potion that Tristan and Isolde unwittingly drank. The symptoms displayed by the immortal lovers were examined in detail, and a theory was developed that the love potion contained herbs from the *Solanaceae* family, especially the thorn-apple (*Datura stramonium*) and deadly nightshade (*Atropa belladonna*), and maybe also traces of monkshood (*Aconitum napellus*) and betony (*Stachys officinalis*). The first two are rich in atropine, hyoscyamine and scopolamine — in other words, alkaloids that paralyze the sympathetic nerve endings of the autonomic nervous system. And that is the sort of intoxication our heroes must have suffered. The effect of these alkaloids on the human organism was known long before the discovery of the autonomic nervous system, and in Renaissance times belladonna was used by Venetian beauties to make their pupils larger and to make their eyes sparkle. Yet we might feel a sort of professional wince at this toxicological view of great love, even more so at the explanation of Isolde's death as being caused by chronic alkaloid poisoning. For it is possible to die — without poison — of longing and despair, as did Tristan's mother, Blanchefleur, after the death of her beloved husband. Thus Isolde's death would be an echo of that death, and the heavily loaded sorrow there at the start of events found its reflection in the name "Tristan." Closer to us than any medical analyses are the words of Thomas Mann, who aptly noted that the great lovers might just as well have drunk a chalice of water, because the potion simply served to make them aware of a love that was already burning with a bright flame.

The story of Tristan and Isolde stirred the imagination of (fortunately!) not only the doctors who tried to find the formula for the love potion, but also some composers. Can timeless love that does not end when life ends be expressed in music? Richard Wagner took on the attempt in his opera *Tristan and Isolde*. It is usually said that he achieved new, striking effects, using the "Tristan chord," that is, a half-diminished seventh chord (or augmented sixth, f-b-d#-g#), whose tonal identity tends to be especially ambiguous. But this interval can also be found in earlier composers — Bach himself used it dozens of times. So the secret must lie elsewhere. At the very start of the work, the emotional intensity is reflected in transitional chromatic notes stretched out one after another, developing step by step. In Bach the augmented sixth resolves into a perfect cadence. In Wagner it gradually ascends, in sequences, to a dominant seventh and advances onwards. This series, this odyssey of a melody that is continuously under strain, that seeks full resolution but never finds

it, means that it has no end: it becomes a "never ending melody."
Like the love that it eulogizes, and that knows no limits.

This is one of the exceptional, successful examples of music
(consciously, by its original intention), virtually merging with a literary text. For, as a rule, it dissociates itself in the work of its great
composers from any kind of illustrative quality. It continues to be
the most inscrutable art: for the poet it is "the breath of statues,"
for the mathematician "music is a secret arithmetical exercise of the
soul, unaware that it is counting." In essence it eludes descriptions
and definitions. It safeguards its purely musical, immaterial impressions that cannot be transferred to any other class of experiences.
Only youth may be unaware of this, and may eagerly attempt to
grasp its essence, or at least part of it. At my music school we were
encouraged to go to concerts at the Krakow Philharmonic. In the
first class, equipped with a school entry pass, I attended a recital by
Arturo Benedetti Michelangeli. From that evening onwards, whenever I walked past a music shop, I thought: "Maybe I'll find his new
recording?," and as I ran my eyes over the concert programs in various cities around the world, I secretly hoped I would see his name,
and that I would go and hear him again. Thus my school instilled a
sense of longing in me before I had yet understood that anticipating a recurrence, such as the recurrence of a musical motif, which is
really nothing other than longing, belongs to the essence of music.

Sometimes it is also true that, at the moment when the enchantment
of love hits us, when we fall in love irrevocably, as the feeling crys-
tallizes within us — we can hear music. And these two simultaneous
occurrences merge inside us and become inseparable. So it was, at
dinner at Madame Verdurin's, that Swann fell in love with Odette,
as the young pianist played a sonata by Vinteuil in the salon. He
had heard it once before, a year ago, at a party, when its leading

motif, a musical phrase, had instantly bewitched him with the sensuous charm of its tones, and when it appeared again, he recognized its line, its shape, and felt a passionate desire to hear it again, once more. At the time this phrase had aroused an extraordinary thrill in him that he had never experienced before. It told him that his life could change, and "he had been filled with love for it as with a new and strange desire." He had looked for it, trying to find out about the work and the composer—in vain, until finally he forgot about it. And when a year later at Madame Verdurin's he suddenly heard it, he was deeply moved and began to tell Odette how he had fallen in love with this phrase, without realizing that he was already telling her about his love for her. From then on this elusive phrase, like something from another world, retained for them its special, irreplaceable charm, the one and only wisdom that "love is all there is." And once he had heard it many times, Swann continued to long for it, even in the later agonies of his love, when he was torn apart by jealousy over Odette, justified jealousy, and then again, when he started to sense that his feelings for her were going cold. For he knew that the longed-for musical phrase would bring back to him "the special, elusive essence of lost happiness—the precise moment of the birth of love."

What about betrayal, the poison of love? Is it really inscribed into human nature? The story of the water nymph, Ondine, is about betrayal. Born in a crystal palace at the bottom of the ocean, she abandons her freedom and life among the waves and makes for the world of people in search of love. The sea current carries her to the shore, where a fisherman and his wife take her in at their cottage, like a gift from heaven. It is there that one day she meets a young knight who has lost his way in the woods by the sea. She falls in love with him at first sight, and it is requited. From then on "for her, loneliness begins two paces away from him." The king of the sea, her uncle, agrees to their wedding, on one condition. He tells Ondine: "If he betrays you, he will die, and you will lose all memory of him forever." Although for her time does not pass—she is always fifteen years old and radiates the natural brightness of a being from another world—she ends up experiencing the fate of a human being. She matures along with her love, coming to know its frenzy and torment, including the cruelest pain of all: betrayal. And then, still in love, she tries to take the blame for her beloved on herself. But the ruler of the sea kingdom knows no mercy: "He who breaks his sacred vow / Woe is he, his life is woe / And woe betide his wicked soul." There is no going back on a bond. At night, while asleep, the knight "forgets to breathe" and dies, and at the same moment Ondine forgets him, forgets her great emotion, the absolute love that she sought in vain among mankind, and returns to her underwater world.

The story of Ondine, which comes from Scandinavian-Germanic myths, was popularized by the German romantic Friedrich de la Motte-Fouqué. There are echoes of it in Mickiewicz, who wrote: "Rumor has it that Ondines appear on the shores of Lake Świteź, in other words, water nymphs, whom the local peasantry call Świtezianki." The story also inspired Claude Debussy and Jean Giraudoux, and finally in the late twentieth century it began to interest many doctors too, including me. Some years ago a mother reported to our clinical ward with her seventeen-year-old son. She had traveled from the other end of Poland, driven by a concern that had come to her in a dream. She had dreamed that her son, as she put it, "had forgotten to breathe in the night and had never woken up again." We knew from her that as soon as he was born, the boy had lain in hospital for six months, probably because of encephalitis, which had passed without trace. Recently he had dropped his girlfriend and was spending nights away from home. Within the family they had never forgotten about a child who had died during apnea. Short pauses in breathing while asleep that last only a few seconds are familiar to medicine. They result from a temporary occlusion of the upper airways; certain features of stature, such as a short neck, obesity or the coexistence of other illnesses can cause a predisposition to it. But the boy definitely did not belong to this category. Apart from the vague history from his babyhood, he had not suffered any brain disease that could have caused sleep disturbances, and the electrocardiogram (ECG) we performed at once excluded the possibility of any unusual family arrhythmia that could have stopped his heart, and after it his breathing. The electroencephalogram was all right too, and so were the neurological tests. We dug out some fat, learned tomes from the library and started casting our suspicions at "Ondine's curse" — an extremely rare, recently identified mystery disorder of the sleep center in the brain, in which a cessation of breathing can come about in the night. None of us had ever seen or heard of an illness like it before. There were no particular ways of diagnosing it, and in our books the only advice we could find was to apply brain stimulants, which just in case we did. For the first few nights we had a nurse sitting by the boy's bed (polysomnography had not yet been invented), and when nothing major happened, we connected him to an ECG monitor linked to an alarm system. One night, there was a storm raging over Krakow, and the electricity was switched off in our district. The hospital, which could not afford a backup generator, was plunged into darkness for two hours. When the lights came back on, the monitors returned to life, and across the screen by our patient's bed ran a straight horizontal line. The boy had stopped breathing in his sleep — and was dead. And we were left with questions that have kept coming back to me for years. What did we fail to do that could have prevented this young death? Insert a tube into him and connect him to a respirator, on the basis of nothing but his mother's dream and an unclear history recurring in the family? (Assisted breathing was not yet known about then.) Maybe instead of trusting electronics, we should have let his mother keep watch over him at night, as she had requested? And this thought occurs, as if through a fog: could it be that Ondine had come back, looking for love in the world of men again? And could she have chosen this very boy, who had proved unfaithful and let her down?

The bedridden patient, unable to move and wracked by suffering, becomes withdrawn, shut in, as within the four walls of the hospital room. The world goes drab and gray, recedes and disappears. Someone who might be able to restore its colors for him and reveal its beauty is a nurse. In *Slow Man* by J.M. Coetzee, a retired photographer named Paul loses a leg in a street accident, which dramatically changes his life. A declared loner, who has never loved or hated, who has in fact been married, but soon divorced, and is childless, he becomes dependent on the help and care of a nurse named Marijana. It is she who brings long-forgotten emotion, concern and femininity into his life. Paul falls in love with the nurse — a simple, warm Croatian girl, "whose sex appeal relies on the fact that as a wife and mother her life is brimming with love," in harmony with the world. The patient experiences an emotion that seems to him sinful and devoid of prospects. His unrequited but very strong feelings prompt questions to occur to him that define us all, questions about the meaning of life, about doing good deeds and about the role of love. And although in the final part, as if embarrassed by the beautiful, dispassionate sentimentality of his story, Coetzee defuses the pathos and forces his hero to laugh at his own tragedy. It is not just the image of a Western man plunged into the depths of egoism, who has forgotten he can love, that remains with us. We are also left with the birth of an emotion that is capable of obscuring pain and illness.

When he had already finished the ninety-first year of his life, Czesław Miłosz spent some time in our hospital because of prolonged episodes of unconsciousness. When on the fourth day of his treatment I visited him early in the morning, he suddenly came to, opened his eyes, smiled happily and said in Polish: "But what pretty *nursy* you have here, Doctor." He used the English word "nurses," but with a Polish grammatical ending. His words had run together as if from two areas of his brain, from the two languages in which he lived, to meet in his first clear, but unexpected sentence for several days. In answer to the smile that moved across his gloomy face like a ray of sunshine, John Keats would probably have responded with a smile of his own, seeing his words come true in it: "yes, in spite of all, / Some shape of beauty moves away the pall / From our dark spirits." Because beauty is the promise of happiness. "Professor," I said, "I have nothing more to do here. I'm going to see the sick patients—you are quite well." I do not know if he heard me; in fact, I think he had fallen asleep again, but he left me with the image of his fleeting, happy smile.

Where might the seat of love be located? We will probably say in the heart. There is no organ in our bodies whose anatomy is better known than the heart, yet no such center has ever been found in it. What if we take an acceptable analogy and ask about the center of the aesthetic pleasures that art brings us? Should we look for it in the brain? Nabokov firmly believed it was between the shoulder blades. He wrote: "That little shiver behind is quite certainly the highest form of emotion that humanity has attained when evolving pure art and pure science. Let us worship the spine and its tingle. Let us be proud of our being vertebrates, for we are vertebrates tipped at the head with a divine flame. The brain only continues the spine: the wick really goes through the whole length of the candle."

And on this aesthetic vibration he added: "If we are not capable of enjoying that shiver, if we cannot enjoy literature, then let us give up the whole thing."

Music can be a source of similar somatic impressions. In a prestigious scientific journal, some Canadian neurologists recently described the research they had done on a group of trained music lovers and musicians who felt shudders and shivers down their spines when they heard their favorite compositions. The experiment fulfilled all the scientific rigors: identical observations were conducted while listening to "indifferent" music that left the audience unmoved. A short piece of music previously found to trigger this mysterious shudder along the spine was accompanied by a faster heartbeat, accelerated breathing, changes in the electrical charges in the muscles and a remarkable arousal of certain centers in the brain. At these moments fresh streams of blood were being sent to the major nuclei of the brain stem, and especially to the structures of the hippocampus, and thus to places where the "pleasure centers" are located in the brain. It seems as if the same clusters of brain cells become aroused and start to radiate a powerful energy when a hungry man gets a slice of bread, a drug addict his hashish or a man who is pining for love gets a woman.

The search for the center of artistic pleasures, and also for the essence of strong aesthetic emotion, is fascinating, "although," as Adam Zagajewski writes, "surely deep in our hearts we all dream of never finding this mysterious something so that we can remain in uncertainty." Because rationalizing a piece of art could be the end of all the fun, a drastic impoverishment of a work "in which the blood of mystery circulates, as the ends of its vessels flow into the surrounding night, to return from there filled with dark fluid." And so in the natural or medical sciences we try unconditionally "to reach a single, empirical answer, but in the humanities we seek one that borders on artistry, not an unambiguous result at all." We want the magic of the mystery, the capacity to be "in uncertainties, mysteries, doubts, without any irritable reaching after fact and reason."

The doctor tries to keep death at bay. He writes prescriptions for longevity in which he mitigates the calorie restrictions with a glass of red wine. But love has its ways and means too. The moving conviction that great love not only continues after death but can even postpone death has persisted through the centuries. We find the origins of this belief in the Greek myth of Alcestis, wife of King Admetus, who is destined to die young. For Apollo, who is the king's friend, Ananke makes an exception: death will accept a substitute for Admetus. And so yet again Apollo stands up to death, which he has already had to conquer once before, in another myth, when he plucked Asclepius from the womb of Coronis as she lay burning on a pyre. But this time it is even harder. He gains Ananke's consent, but no one is eager to give up their life for the king, even though he is a just, popular ruler. All his relatives and friends refuse, and so do his old mother and old father. Death is already approaching, and mocks Apollo, saying to him, as Ted Hughes puts it: "What you call death is simply my natural power, / The pull of my gravity. And life / is a brief weightlessness—an aberration / From the status quo—which is me." So too was Admetus's life, and you cannot help, death triumphantly declares, not even you, Apollo, the healer-god:

> Life is your hospital and you call it a funfair,
> Your silly sickroom screen of giggling faces,
> Your quiver full of hypodermic syringes
> That you call arrows of inspiration.
> Man is deluded and his ludicrous gods
> Are his delusion. Death is death is death.

And then a substitute for Admetus comes forward. She volunteers of her own accord, as no one has dared approach her. It is Alcestis, his beautiful wife, who refuses to live a single day without her beloved husband. For her, that would be greater suffering than death. And so death takes her down to Hades. But once again it is forced to relinquish a dead person when Heracles appears and rescues Alcestis. In the final scene he returns her to her husband, who is already plunged into mourning. This scene would probably have lacked force of expression, and should even have fallen flat, if only because of the none-too-convincing Admetus, who from the start sees nothing inappropriate in the idea of his wife dying for his sake and instead of him. So it probably would have, if not for Euripides's brilliant ingenuity. (But I had better let him tell you about it himself, Reader!) And so this unusual story has a bright and happy ending.

The Greeks doubted that a woman was capable of feeling *philia* towards a man — "that friendship which grows out of love ... and which only men were supposed to experience." But Alcestis was capable of it. She knew of no higher value than love, and she was willing to sacrifice herself for it. So it is no surprise that on seeing this, the gods agreed that Heracles could return her to life and release her from Hades. This story inspired not only poets but also musicians, and lives on in operas by Lully, Handel and Gluck. In an altered state, it has even gone into the future, into the world of cloned human beings described in *Never Let Me Go*, a novel by Kazuo Ishiguro, where in the depths of their memory the clones have preserved the myth of a death sentence deferred by love.

Paracelsus knew about the power of love and never tried to cure it. We will find no such remedy in his monumental work, *The Archidoxes of Magic*, published for the first time, posthumously, in Krakow in 1569, and a year later in five other European cities. Yet it contains an abundant list of drugs, a quasi–prescription book, thanks to which its author is regarded as the father of chemotherapy, in other words, of treating illnesses with chemical drugs. Others thought of it before him, but he was the most ardent and influential proponent of this idea, which in the seventeenth century changed the course of medical thinking. However, even in writing about "laudanum," he never recommends using it to treat love sickness. Yet this was his peerless drug, ultra-powerful against the most difficult illnesses, a true elixir that was even supposed to awaken the dead. It is wrongly assumed that laudanum was a narcotic extracted from poppy seeds. A year ago, at the "Piwnica Pod Baranami" cabaret in Krakow, I heard Tamara Kalinowska singing in a dreamy voice a song called *A Drop of Laudanum for Every Day*, playfully turning to look at me as she sang the final verse:

> *Try it in the forearms by skilful injection,*
> *The Doctor could join the Magician's domain,*
> *Do it in the washroom avoiding detection,*
> *A small dose of laudanum into the vein.*

The cabaret was not the best place to straighten out the false reputation of laudanum, or at least laudanum as Paracelsus understood it. So I kept quiet, knowing, however, that the great doctor and magician in one person was familiar with and used opiates made of poppy seed, and gave them explicit names, without confusing them with laudanum. There is no way of ascertaining what Paracelsus's laudanum was, because he writes about it vaguely and mysteriously, sometimes implying that he manufactured it, using extremely precious ingredients, not excluding gold and pearls. Some have even reckoned it was a metaphysical concept, a sort of healing principle. Nothing we can find in Paracelsus's writings brings us any closer to an explanation of this enigma. Some have called his work "unintelligible ravings"; others have enthused that they are "admirably clear." It is not hard to discern contradictions in his words, and a desire to prompt recognition and admiration; he uses neologisms to hide from mockery and rejection, and he fears the reader's indifference. Carried away by inspiration, he took no notice of the details. His work and life are pervaded by an original vision of Nature — "his vision of nature was so grand and weaves so fine and so dense a net that it is hard to pull on one strand without awakening all the others." Before his eyes he had "a magical image of the universe, distilled in the red-hot alembic of his fevered imagination."

This medical wizard who cured eighteen kings and princes when all the doctors had abandoned them, this solitary, tireless and obstreperous nomad, who eagerly sought medicinal knowledge in experience, enjoys unflagging interest to this day. Every year new books and scholarly articles about him appear. He perceived the entire world through an original concept that is the foundation of his medicine, stating that man harmonizes with the cosmos. Illness was a breach of this accord, a dissonance. The task of a doctor was to restore the broken harmony and attune the patient to the rhythms of the universe. That medical theme was written into his entire philosophy, representing "man's original and specific mission ... he has been placed in the world solely for this purpose." In creating the world, says Paracelsus, God did not imprison it in a closed form of perfection, but left the road to development open before it. Man's task is to follow that road and shape himself and the world with a view to perfection. He was in no doubt that the *ars magna*, alchemy, was this Royal Way. Through persistent attempts at transmuting matter and spirit — from the inferior to the superior — the alchemists strove towards their own perfection. The mysteries of the secret art were meant to liberate them from the confinement of their own skins, raise them upwards and unite them with the cosmos. In this sense Paracelsus took part in the transmutation of the world and continued the work of creation.

As John Paul II reminds us, after the Book of Genesis, "all men and women are entrusted with the task of crafting their own life: in a certain sense, they are to make of it a work of art, a masterpiece." Here we have an echo of the idea that the work of creation is not finished. It is still going on, and in some sense we ourselves are the distant continuers of the divine breath (*ruah*) with which the Holy Spirit pervades the world, just as it did at its origin. Because, asked Rainer Maria Rilke, what would be the sense of our journey through life, into the future, if He, whom we seek, belonged to the past? Might we not suppose He will come after all, and will contain everything? And in an enchanting comparison, he said: "As bees collect honey, so we take what is sweetest out of everything and build Him. We start actually with the slight, with the unpretentious (if only it is done with love) ... Is there anything which can take from you the hope of thus being hereafter in him, in the most distant, the uttermost?" These inspired words speak of the creative power of love. Only love can liberate us from the tyranny of the "Self." The omnipotent *ego* falls silent as we stand dazzled in an altered world. We are no longer living for ourselves alone.

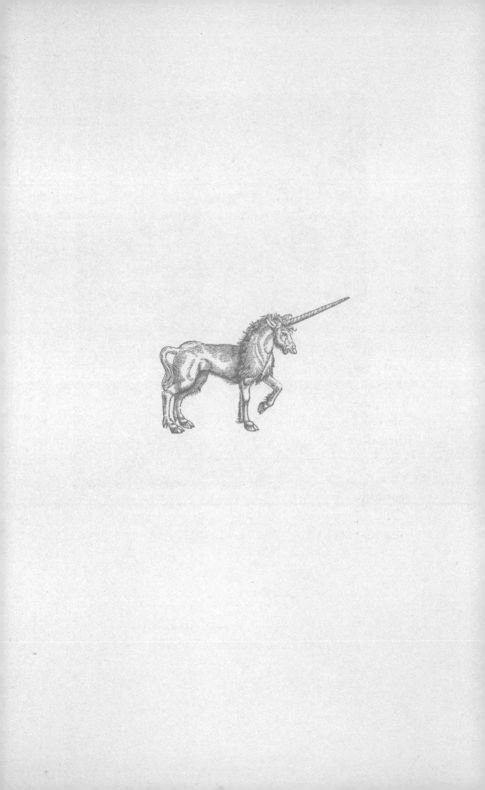

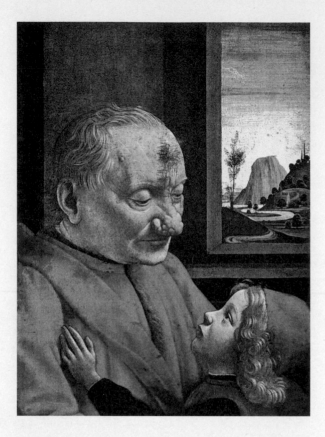

Domenico Ghirlandaio
An Old Man and His Grandson, c. 1490
Louvre, Paris

CONJUNCTION

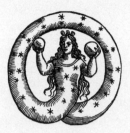

In the final years of his life, Francisco Goya painted many portraits of his friends. He created them quickly, at a single sitting, with broad strokes of his brush. "My eye does not perceive features or details," he admitted. "I do not count the hairs in the beard of a man walking past me, and the buttonholes in his coat do not hold my gaze. My brush cannot see any more than I can."

In 1819, when he reached the age of seventy-three, he fell dangerously ill and came close to death. A year later he painted his stunning *Self-Portrait with Doctor Arrieta* (*Goya curado por el doctor Arrieta*). In it he expressed his gratitude to the man in whom he placed boundless trust and who had saved his life. The picture was provided with a long inscription, on the model of the ones placed by votive offerings hanging in Spanish churches to give thanks for miraculous intervention in times of trouble. The doctor and friend of the artist proved to be a *curandero* (healer) of a very different kind from the *matasanos*—the killers of healthy people, the quack doctors whom Goya had always ridiculed with his brush. In the picture the artist has depicted himself with full sincerity: he is sitting in bed with his head drooping, his face is puffy, his eyes are half-closed and his lips are clenched. You can almost hear how heavily he is breathing. Death must have been close by, because the patient's hands are convulsively gripping the bedclothes. The doctor is leaning over his patient with an arm around him as he raises a glass of medicine to his lips and gently makes him drink. Doctor Arrieta's face shows gravity and concern, but also strong emotion. "His embrace is stronger than the grip of death." In the dark background loom three figures. Are they gawkers, relatives or phantoms from the other world? Looking at the portrait, it is hard to believe that Goya still had an entire powerful cycle of "Black Paintings" ahead of him, and some very creative years in Bordeaux. However we explain the enigmas of the painting, it emanates affection; life is winning against death — this time.

At the moment captured in the painting, the doctor and his patient are living as one. Their lives were connected, united. The ancient Greeks would have said they were in symbiosis. This word appears for the first time in Theophrastus, a pupil of Aristotle and author of an illustrious treatise on botany entitled *On the Causes of Plants*. There we find the sentence: "As for a plant's growing on trees and other plants when it also grows in the earth, there is no oddity . . ." No; the oddity is that a plant grows exclusively on another plant, and not on the ground. Now it may perhaps be that, like animals, plants are fond of one another and *live together* (σύμβιος). The word, "symbiosis," which was derived from biology, soon found a place in literary and colloquial language. Aristotle writes about "the need for people as *companions for coexistence* (*symbiosis*) and on rendering them kindnesses." Others follow in his footsteps — Isocrates, Polybius and Diodorus Siculus, and Antipater of Tarsus even introduces symbiosis into the title of his treatise *On Life with a Woman*

(*Peri ginaikos simbioscos*). For the Greeks, symbiosis must have sounded clear and obvious. The particle *sym-* plainly determined a connection, evoking "symphony," "sympathy," "symposium," "symmetry," and dozens of other words in which for phonetic reasons it underwent modification to *syn-*, while retaining its strength of meaning ("synonym," "synthesis," "synergy," etc.). The popular spread of the term "symbiosis" was also promoted by Theophrastus's literary talent. Two thousand years later he provided an abundant source for La Bruyère, who copied his style as well as his structure. In biology, however, the term passed into oblivion, to return in its precise meaning only at the end of the nineteenth century. Biologists pedantically differentiate the reactions that take place between organisms, using terms to describe so-called non-antagonistic relations such as "mutualism," "commensalism" and others, for example. The overriding concept of symbiosis occupies a special place of its own. We came across it in the first stages of the origin and development of life, in discussing endosymbiosis. A protozoan such as *Paramecium bursaria* contains five genomes at once: its own nucleus and its own mitochondria, and, in addition, endosymbiotic chlorophytes, each of which contains its own nucleus, its own mitochondria and its own chloroplasts. "And so this microscopic organism that uses its cilia to row its way across the great gulf of a drop of water performs the functions—in one phenotype—of five genotypes at once." Fat volumes on biology and ecology are entirely filled with chapters on symbiosis, because this sort of coexistence is one of the most common forms of life. Thanks to the combination of mycelia and algae, lichens are prevalent in polar and mountain tundra, growing on rocks, concrete and the bark of trees, and there are at least fourteen thousand varieties of them. Almost all herbivorous animals take advantage of symbiotic organisms living inside them—protozoa, fungi and bacteria—to be able to digest cellulose, the most abundant source of energy on Earth.

We too carry bacteria in our intestines, and in astronomical numbers. In an era when hygiene is so dominant, the knowledge that there are a hundred trillion bacteria living in the digestive tract of each one of us comes as a shock. Although they do not serve us, as they do herbivores, to assimilate cellulose, in fact they provide ten percent of all the energy absorbed in the intestines, and they produce important nutrients, such as vitamin K. It remains a mystery how our immune system peacefully coexists with such a vast legion of microbes.

If using the word "symbiosis" to describe the connection between doctor and patient smacks too much of biology for you, Reader, or takes the contact too close, you can replace it with the word "conjunction." Then the associations shift from biology to astronomy and logic, and they are less permanent in nature, at least in relation to the heavenly bodies. The connection will not come about, much less grow strong, without the patient's trust. On the doctor's part it simply comes down to remembering the patient, thinking about him and keeping him in mind. And so to the question, "What should the doctor know about the patient?" I reply: "All about his illness, and quite a lot about him." By this I mean that if he were shaken awake in the middle of the night, the doctor should at once be able to rattle off the anamnesis and the test results of any patient he is caring for in the hospital ward. I expect this of the junior colleagues who work with me, and woe betide them if I catch them not knowing the facts. (You see what a joy it is to work with me, Reader!) But otherwise there is no medicine. Of course there is a health service, a National Health Fund and even a Ministry of Health—but no medicine.

Aren't these expectations excessive, or even idealized? I don't think so. Let us take an example from science. The eminent physicist Andrzej Białas says that his mentor, Professor Jan Weyssenhoff, taught him "the most important thing, namely, that you think about physics nonstop. Day and night." He was able to do this as soon as he fell under the spell of the beauty of physics, as demonstrated by his mentor. Not to mention the effects of the spell of love — in the margins of his inspired sketches for his great paintings, Raphael wrote sonnets to La Fornarina.

Why is it so hard to "be with a sick person"? Because loyalty is not one of the strongest features of human nature, and there are all sorts of obstacles, starting from the mundane, such as tiredness, family obligations or putting personal pleasures above duty. Low salaries increase haste, and the need for a second or third paying job. And on top of that, there is the ever-growing bureaucracy and its inescapable machinery; the unwise instructions of the European Union, which regulates a doctor's work hours in such a way that there is a different doctor taking care of the patients in a hospital each day; and the commercialism of medicine, the consequence of abruptly rising costs of treatment. The avalanche of costs is burying health care. Richer countries than ours are battling with this problem, although it seems as if the accumulation of ills is especially large in Poland. Hence there are strict controls on expenditure for treatment and endless financial restrictions. In the contracts for "services" that we sign with the National Health Fund, the word "doctor" is vanishing, to be replaced by "the contractor." Until finally the doctor starts to pay more attention to the economist than to his own conscience.

The public health care system is gradually eroding the mystery of medicine. The doctor's outer skin is getting calloused and he is losing his sensitivity. In Poland, in contrast to the Anglo-Saxon countries, for example, information about the patient following a specialist consultation or hospital treatment is not sent by letter to the family doctor, but is handed to the patient in the form of an information sheet. We always used to write the diagnosis on these sheets, as on the temperature charts hanging by the beds, in Latin. The word "cancer" was never mentioned in full. A single letter stood for it (and even now as I write this, my pen hesitates to use the word). So too the doctors used to talk to each other in a hushed tone by the patient's beds during their rounds, avoiding drastic terms and peppering their sentences with Latin jargon, so that the patient would not take everything literally, would not be terrified and would be saved worry and fear. What is more, his neighbors could hear the conversations, because hospital wards were rarely separate, one-person rooms. Must their fellow sufferers know everything about any particular patient? About intimate matters? In one sense, it is a doctor's task to protect the patient from sudden bad news about his health, especially when it is debatable and not fully proven. These are obvious, human considerations, based on a firm belief in the rightness of sustaining hope.

However, this is changing. To suit the National Health Fund officials who control whether each information sheet following hospital treatment fits properly in their drawers full of signed contracts for "services," the Ministry of Health recently gave instructions for diagnoses to be written in Polish, and in detail, in order to justify the diagnostic procedures performed and the treatment applied. If the patient is going to set eyes on what is quite often devastating news in writing anyway, is there any sense in wrapping it in cotton wool during the general ward round? Why not write it straight onto the temperature chart for all the visitors to see? These checks and restraints are disappearing. And with them sensitivity and the mystery of medicine are also evaporating.

We could ask: should we therefore tell the patient the truth? The question is badly put. The answer to it is: of course we should.

But we should also ask: how are we to tell that truth? The doctor's sensitivity and personality traits come to light right at these critical moments when we have to approach the truth, and the truth may be terrible. Does a sick person really want to hear the entire truth? Even when he says: "I know I have cancer. I am prepared for anything; please tell me the truth," his eyes say something different: "Tell me the truth I want to hear; give me some hope."

The patient should not suddenly hear the whole, cruel truth from the doctor. It blinds and kills hope. And we all carry hope inside us. It is a powerful force that allows us to face up to illness. Moreover, it has deeper and deeper biological foundations. Medicine can provide proof of close connections between the nervous system and the immune system. We are starting to understand why psychological shock can break down resistance, and why for centuries people have collapsed when struck by dreadful news. Hope is integral to the medical calling. As Petronius said: *Medicus enim nihil aliud est quam animi consolatio* — "The doctor is nothing more than consolation for the soul."

If the truth can be a poison, it should be applied in small doses, like chemotherapeutic anti-cancer drugs, which if applied in too high a dose can also kill. These things are never discussed at medical school, nor do they come up in specialist exams. Yet they are the doctor's daily bread, and they — as well as philosophical and ethical attitudes — affect the course and results of treatment. In my view, the way a doctor conveys the truth, the style he uses, is decisive. And the time — he has to find the time to share the patient's journey, leading to a revelation of the truth. Must he always follow it right to the very end, from where he can see all the consequences of the illness without exception? That depends on the patient's sensitivity, psychological makeup, family and life situation. The arcana of the art should help the doctor to evaluate them, so that he can mobilize them to fight for the patient's health.

In revealing the truth to the patient, we do not forget to be in touch with the family, with someone who is close to him, one or two people perhaps. But what should we do if all of a sudden dozens of them appear? When I was a young doctor, one day I was walking to my department across the hospital garden. That was what we called, with considerable exaggeration, the square patch of grass in the courtyard surrounded by the neo-Gothic red-brick buildings housing the university departments. That morning it was covered in tents and wagons, with horses let loose to nibble the grass. Sparks were shooting from a bonfire under a cauldron hanging on a low tripod. A large gypsy camp had been set up in the usually empty courtyard. The night before their queen had appeared at our department, the wife of the King of the Gypsies from the Kwiek family.

They flew down unexpectedly, as at Macondo, in the southern hemisphere. But Melquiades was not among them, who would have given an impressive display of something he himself called the eighth wonder of the world, invented by the learned alchemists of Macedonia. No, he was not there to show us the magical magnets that could free metal objects from immobility, proving that they live their own life: "it's simply a matter of waking up their souls." Our gypsies never even peeped inside the hospital, but just camped out in the square day after day. They were simply there. At first shyly, and then in larger and larger numbers, the patients began to visit them. And the swarthy, handsome gypsy women, wrapped in long shawls, with children in their arms or clinging to their skirts, told the patients the future from cards. The men traded or quietly played music. The smoke of the bonfire was carried on the wind, and with it came mysterious gusts of something foreign and unusual, ". . . as if a gate had been left open in the usual life, as if something might get in or get out." And one night, through this gate they vanished. The queen had recovered and left the hospital, so they had flown away with her like birds — to the *romano drom*, the gypsy road.

Gradually, we returned to normal life, to puzzling out the riddles. For the doctor, each patient is a riddle. The riddle is solved when a diagnosis is reached. It is no simple matter, though it is one of the most important medical skills. You have to hear the patient out, while steering the conversation to extract the most important symptoms of the illness from him; you have to know how to spot and investigate their hallmarks and finally you have to enrich the whole process with additional tests, laboratory or imaging ones, for example. During this complex procedure, we never stop considering myriad diagnoses as we narrow the circle of suspects and separate the chaff from the grain. We make this journey with the patient, explaining the point of each diagnostic step. Finally, the time comes to tell him the diagnosis and decide on the treatment. At this point, certain essential traits of the doctor's personality come together. God forbid he should show features of paternalism, a practice that has been picked to shreds in recent decades. This is the attitude of a father figure, who worries about his children's welfare without taking their views into account. This is a benevolent but authoritarian approach to the patient. It is at odds with the emancipation imperative — the modern tendency to free us from our social, cultural and even biological roles. Paternalism ignores or limits the patient's autonomy, and by doing so it removes his partnership and conscious involvement in his own treatment.

Criticism of authoritarianism has promoted other models for the doctor-patient relationship. In the consumer model the doctor is the seller of medical services, just like any other commercial services on the free market. He is meant to be neutral. He can give advice but should not influence the decisions — it is the patient who decides what to choose and what to buy from the medical supermarket. He "would become a purchaser of services and often would be referred to as a client." In the negotiation model, which concludes with a contract, each side tries to gain advantages at the other's expense. The patient aims to obtain those advantages at the lowest price. The doctor, conversely, tries to exclude risky solutions whose failure would end in a lawsuit, a verdict and compensation. Thus the doctor will be less concerned about a proper cure for the patient and more about legally fulfilling the contractual demands. This model dehumanizes the doctor-patient relationship and is at odds with the medical vocation.

Although disapproval of paternalism has rightly highlighted the patient's role and his freedom, it has also brought losses. In extreme cases it has turned into a dispute between competing egotistical liberties — the patient's and the doctor's. Yet the autonomy of both the one and the other must be subordinate to the good of the patient. It is not his autonomy but the person that is the absolute value. A person's dignity should not be reduced to nothing but his liberty, because worthy as well as unworthy human behavior can result from liberty. And there is no better plane for achieving the full benefit to the patient than mutual trust. That is what builds interpersonal bonds, and it includes liberty among the values that it achieves. An environment of trust is a therapeutic environment. "It builds a sphere of safety for the patient." It builds his faith in people.

At this point should we not discuss, or at least mention, the features of a doctor that guarantee a proper relationship with his patients, ensuring a bond and trust? The answer is negative, for two reasons. The number of desirable values and virtues could easily stretch into an almost endless stream that would take the doctor close to the realm of angels. Bombarded as he is with news about bribe taking and corruption among doctors, the Polish reader would be entitled to think that I am writing like a mathematician describing a world of unreal numbers. The plague of dishonesties — which exists in other countries too, though rarely to such an extent as in Poland — should, of course, be dealt with in the public prosecutor's office. And the second reason: It would be a pity to encapsulate the answer in a single formula or example, as the wealth of proper reactions, behavior and deeds is immense. For the young trainee in the art of medicine, his model will be his mentor, and there is nothing more important — at this period in his training — than finding him. And on reading these words, let the patient remember the doctor whom he liked so much that he trusted him without hesitation. In every case there will be examples of this, though all slightly different.

Let us also raise the significance of the singular here, because "where many cure, no one cures" (*Quod multi curant, nemo curat*). "Man is not an aggregate," in which the individual elements are subject to separate laws or fields of science that describe and improve them. For the psyche "aggregate" there are psychologists, for the social life there are sociologists, the spiritual one, priests, and of course there is a different medical specialist for each internal organ. Although the refined art of the individual specialist might convince us that the patient can easily be dismantled into his component parts, each of which will be cleaned up and fixed, then put back together to function perfectly, in fact the role of a single person to coordinate and harmonize all these activities is crucial. This is true for complicated cases, and in simple ones the doctor should be driven by the ambition to square up to the illness and get rid of it.

✦✦✦

The doctor's vocation and the relationship between physician and patient is described to us in the writings of Hippocrates, the founder of medical ethics within the traditions of Western medicine. To this day, on completing their studies medical students take a solemn vow to keep the principles contained in the Hippocratic oath. It is regarded as a timeless, synthetic record of the ethical standards required of doctors. It is a short list, "consisting of nine elaborate sentences." It includes invocations defining the relationship of the person taking the oath to his teacher and to the art (of medicine), and the general principles of medical conduct. But an oath is not really suitable, because it cannot respond to many of the specific but essential problems of modern medicine. Take the first to hand, which is a well-publicized example: stem cells. The expectations and hopes that are placed in them are huge. They have been stirred up by the daily press, the scientists and doctors themselves, sick people and their families. This faith in the healing power of stem cells — with a distant view to reproductive cloning — derives from the Promethean ambitions that have accompanied man throughout his history. But does using the noble though still remote idea of helping the sick as an excuse really leave us free to interfere with human embryos at the earliest stages of their development? Even the legislation in different countries varies diametrically on this issue, from a total ban to complete liberalism. Not only could these issues have been unknown to Hippocrates, but they are also unfamiliar to middle-aged doctors in practice today. And what about the question of death and the prolonged coma in a vegetative state lasting for months on end that can precede it? And demands being made for euthanasia? How is a doctor to behave?

Finding a clear answer is complicated by increasingly relative concepts and fluid meanings, as reflected in postmodern art. If the meaning of the concept of truth is questioned and is falling apart, while uncritical pluralism, calling itself tolerance, is proclaiming that all views have identical worth, then where are we to find a foothold? How easy it is to get bogged down in the shifting sands of universal relativism. Yet in the medical profession we are dealing with ethical matters on a daily basis — it is impossible to avoid them. Sometimes everyday life brings a specific answer to issues debated by ethicists and philosophers. In Poland we experienced this quite recently in a case of attempted euthanasia.

In 2007 Poland's first petition for euthanasia reached the courts. It was made by J.Ś., a thirty-two-year-old man who since an accident at the age of fourteen had been paralyzed from the neck down. He was asking for his respirator to be switched off. In justification he plainly insisted that he wanted to go on living only as long as his parents were alive. It was clear that once they were no longer able to take care of him, he would be left entirely alone. The relevant services showed very little interest, the local social aid centers were a disappointment and apparently so were the local parishes and neighbors. The disabled man's letter was a shocking cry of despair. It was not a petition for death, but the call for help of a man who was suffering, abandoned, left completely unaided, because his very old, exhausted parents were looking after him. "We should be hearing hundreds of thousands more cries of this kind, from people who are shut in mental hospitals, but should not be there. I am thinking, for example, of autistic people who are dying of hypostatic pneumonia because they are rotting away in hospitals, chained to their beds, or of abandoned, handicapped people for whom there is less and less room in society," wrote Sister Małgorzata Chmielewska, an exceptional person, who heads the *Chleb życia* ("Bread of Life") community that runs homes for homeless, sick single mothers and night shelters for men and women.

A couple of weeks after the sick man's petition to the court appeared in the daily papers, we read the following headline: "J.Ś. has forgotten about death; he wants to live." Reading onwards, we learned that he had finally started to smile, because people had shown him interest and support, which for years he had never dreamed possible. But to return to an active way of life and feel needed, he wanted to work. What can someone do if only his mind is able, but he needs other people to help him? He gave his own answer to this question: "I can talk. No one is better at comforting and finding a way out of a hopeless situation. I have already been through everything imaginable. I have been to the wall and bounced off it." The priceless Anna Dymna and her foundation for the disabled, *Mimo wszystko* ("In Spite of All"), immediately gave him a job and organized a nationwide telephone connection for him. Efforts to get him a wheelchair were also successfully completed. It had become clear that in asking for death he had been crying out for life, and now, only a few weeks later, he was bursting into this new life.

In this particular case, can we speak of artificially sustaining life? J.Ś. is undoubtedly alive thanks to medical equipment, but "for God's sake, what did we invent it for?!" The whole concept of euthanasia is becoming more and more ambiguous, as shown by the dramatically rising volume of terminology. There is talk of euthanasia, autothanasia, disthanasia, orthothanasia, eugenic, economic and other forms of euthanasia. Passive and active euthanasia are also mentioned, as are direct and indirect, voluntary and involuntary ... This wide variety of terms and debates cannot erase the difference between a natural death and one that is deliberate, forced and induced. The claim that administered death gives the patient his dignity, and a death that is not administered takes it away from him, is "an ethical perversion. It discriminates against all the disabled and suffering people who in the name of their dignity are bravely going through life."

CONJUNCTION

And finally a personal comment. In all my years of medical practice, I have never heard a patient ask for euthanasia. Sister Chmielewska has had the same experience, and yet she has cared for only people who are chronic sufferers and the incurably sick, most of whom "knew their days were numbered. But they also knew they had the support of our love, they were surrounded by it."

What usually suggests the idea of cutting life short is pain. It hacks into us, displaces everything else and takes us over day and night. We know it is an alien force, and "just like a curse, we can only easily utter it in a language not our own." Since time immemorial the forerunners of doctors — sorcerers and shamans — tried to relieve pain, turning to extracts from plants for this purpose. And no other drugs would accompany man more faithfully throughout his history than the ones that soothe pain — the salicylates and opiates. Today there is a very wide range of painkillers, and also of ways to keep taking them. We can stop pain in its tracks and wipe it from our consciousness. Is the ideal we are striving for a life without pain? A small group of young people who lead such a life are a warning to us.

It all began with a ten-year-old boy in northern Pakistan, who used to take part in street performances, sticking knives into his hands or walking on red-hot coals without batting an eyelid. He was one of six children who never felt pain. Their parents did not share this unusual trait. Detailed neurological testing showed that in all six their other senses were perfectly normal. They reacted to touch and pressure, and could tell the difference between alternately applied hot and cold rods, they laughed when they were tickled and they had no trouble sensing the way their bodies were arranged. Everything was in order, except that they were indifferent to pain.

Pain is caused by various stimuli in the special nerve endings for pain that densely cover our body's integument and its insides. These are pain sensors, or receptors or, to use the professional terminology, nociceptors. From them, impulses travel from the periphery along the nerves — like electric trains — to ganglia in the spinal cord and onwards, along its paths, to the brain. And so the signal originates in the specialized receptors or, to be precise, in their cell membranes. They are equipped with small ducts that regulate the flow of ions, and in this way generate a difference of potentials. So, for example, the sodium channels are found in the pain receptors in up to ten forms. The gene controlling one of them — "SCN9A, also known as Nav 1.7," turned out to be mutant in the six Pakistani siblings, and so their receptors were damaged. It was unable to receive sensations of pain. An idea arose of seeking drugs that could block these receptors in normal people. Because there are no such receptors in the heart, or in the central nervous system, pain signals coming from the heart to herald ischemia, such as a heart attack, would remain undisturbed by these hypothetical drugs. The catch is that indifference to pain did not make the Pakistani children healthy — on the contrary, they all had injured lips and tongues, because they had kept biting themselves until the age of four. Some of them had lost the distal parts of their tongues as a result, and others had to undergo plastic surgery. They were covered in bruises and injuries, and easily broke bones. The breaks were complicated to heal, with frequent infections, because the patients, unable to feel pain, did not protect their limbs from movement. So pain, which for us has an invariably negative tinge and is associated with suffering, shows us in this story its other face: as a herald of danger. The pain released by our first defense mechanisms is telling us to stop, making us keep still and directing us to seek help.

◆◆◆

Our life span is getting longer. In the past hundred years we have gained an average twenty-five years. A quarter of a century added to our life! Isn't that the start of a quest for immortality? But we cannot restore youth. And immortality without youth, the Greeks claimed, is a misery. That was their firm belief, which they expressed in mythology, as Michelangelo knew. And on the ceiling of the Sistine Chapel, of the five Sibyls, he gave only one an old face—the Cumaean Sibyl, who obtained immortality from Apollo, but without keeping her youth and beauty. The story of Eos—Aurora, the morning star—also refers to this theme. The poets extolled this beautiful woman, who every day opened the gates of the East, leaped into her chariot of rose petals and crossed the horizon, to send the morning dew down onto Earth and cover the sky in trails of brightness in honor of her brother the Sun. Night and sleep fled from her, and the stars put out their light. Eos was very amorous and had adventures with many of the gods, but her greatest love was the Trojan prince Tithonus. She brought him to Olympus and begged Zeus to give him immortality, which he granted. They lived long and happily, but with time Tithonus began to age, because in asking for his immortality Eos had forgotten to ask for eternal youth. Gradually, before her eyes, he changed into a tiny, shriveled old man. Unable to bear this sight, she shut him in a little wooden box. Eventually, Zeus set him free, changing him into a cicada, and sent him back to Earth. In a seventeenth-century French lithograph we see a beautiful, young, winged Eos leaning over Tithonus, lying under a tree; as she tenderly kisses him farewell, he is already starting to grow an insect's abdomen.

Modern medicine seeks the answers to questions about longevity in genetics. At the molecular level aging involves an accumulation of injuries, defects and fissures in the DNA, which gradually loses its capacity to repair itself. As a result, the pool of stem cells—which are essential for the continuous renewal of multicellular organisms, such as ourselves—dwindles. The source of young, new cells runs dry. This is how we explain aging to ourselves, but we are still a long way from any pharmacological intervention into these extremely complex processes. We are more likely to gain extra years of life from progress in preventing and curing common illnesses, and probably caloric restrictions too. Limiting what we eat by twenty to forty percent (though not suddenly and without descending to malnourishment) seems to lead to a longer life. The proof from the world of animals is convincing, but in humans, there is a need for long-term observation. So how many extra years will we give ourselves? Maybe ten, maybe fifteen, but no one can imagine the average lifespan exceeding one hundred in the next few generations. The limit, though vague, looms somewhere on the horizon.

Things are different for life outside the organism, outside the body, life in vitro, in a test tube. Here immortality appears before our very eyes. The services of Alexis Carrel in this field are impressive. After hearing about successful attempts to cultivate embryonic frog cells, in 1910 to 1912 he developed an original method for cultivating mature human tissues. Although fifty years later his successors mocked this surgeon, who without posing any hypotheses sought and found practical solutions to the problems that fascinated him, and criticized him—rightly so—for the racist views that he expressed towards the end of his life, it was his experimental work that laid the foundations for tissue cultivation. Today it is conducted in thousands of laboratories all over the world. However, he won considerable fame and renown in his lifetime not for his experiments on human tissue, but for his "immortal chicken heart." Carrel took a piece of the heart of a chicken embryo and put it in a glass container. The isolated cells went on beating steadily, outside the organism. By changing the nutritional fluids, which he had tested in advance, keeping it antiseptic and making various minor but crucial improvements, Carrel kept them alive. And they went on beating for a month, a second, and a third—which was reported on the front pages of the newspapers. A heart, the symbol of life and the emotions, which anyone can feel simply by putting a hand to his chest, was now beating on its own—in "a glass pickle jar." It made an immense impression. The experiment fired the imagination of journalists, who wrote about their amazement and wonder, but also horror—"it is like a blood-chilling story by Edgar Allan Poe." The heart of the chicken stopped beating after a hundred and forty days, but the cells in the jar went on dividing and multiplying, although as the months and years went by they changed into fibrous tissue. But the press regularly celebrated the first, the second and then subsequent anniversaries of the "beating chicken heart." And under the influence of Bergson's philosophy, Carrel himself wrote about "life removed from the power of time," about life "outside time," and no longer spoke of "permanent life" but "immortal life," about "immortality."

True in vitro immortality, however, was shown to us by a young woman who in 1951 went to see a doctor at the Johns Hopkins University hospital in Baltimore. She was a black woman named Henrietta Lacks. She sought medical advice because of bleeding from the reproductive tract between periods. A biopsy was performed to establish a diagnosis of cervical cancer. Part of the sample ended up at a small laboratory, where they were trying to cultivate cells with the aim of differentiating various forms of cervical cancer. (Unfortunately, no one asked Henrietta for her opinion or permission.) Her cells amazed the researchers. They were phenomenally lively, and kept multiplying in vitro ad infinitum. They coped perfectly with the hardships of travel, and proved an excellent medium for viruses, including the polio virus, inoculations for which all of America desired at the time. The HeLa cells — as they were named after the patient's initials — were sent from laboratory to laboratory, from one coast of the United States to the other, and later to Europe and the entire world. Henrietta had long since passed on; she died eight months after her diagnosis was established. But part of her is still alive. HeLa cells can be bought from mail order stores selling biological and medical reagents and materials, and tens of thousands of laboratories are working on them worldwide, including my laboratory as I write these words. After more than half a century they are still bursting with the same vigor, the same energy and *élan vital* as on the day they left Henrietta Lacks.

And so life has come out of a body and taken up residence in the glass containers that we have assigned it to. It has proved amazingly plastic, receptive to various experiments and interventions. We are able to freeze it, arrest it in a literal sense by reducing it to a temperature of minus eighty degrees Celsius or lower, preserving it in this state for years, and then, by removing it from the low temperatures, to wake it up, synchronize time for the cells and reanimate them. If we take a piece of skin from a baby guinea pig and freeze it for a year, and then after that time graft it back on again, all our animal's cells will have exactly the same genetic repertoire, but their age will be different. So we will have made the guinea pig into a "time chimera." These and similar experiments are having an increasing influence on our understanding of life and time in biology. If we also knew how to transport a person back in time and turn back the hands of his biological clock, the fate of Henrietta Lacks might have been completely different. The illness that carried her off so quickly is the world's second most common cancer in women. Every year half a million new cases are diagnosed, with eighty percent of the susequent deaths in so-called developing countries. The cancer is caused by a human papilloma virus (HPV) that is sexually transmitted. An effective, prophylactic inoculation has now been produced against the most common strains of this virus, and in mid-2007 the U.S. Centers for Disease Control and Prevention recommended that all girls aged eleven to twelve be inoculated with it. In this way yet another illness is being brought in line, with the prospect of eradicating it entirely in developed countries, and with the hope that the remedy will also reach the continents and countries where this cancer gathers its richest harvest. Although, of course, it is not impossible that the virus, sensing the danger, will start to dodge and weave, mutate and change its shape. Then we shall set off in pursuit of it, with the new inoculations and new anti-viral drugs that we lack today.

Illnesses keep changing, as today's diseases move into the shadows and new ones come into the light. Something tells us we will manage to deal with them. This is surely a product of positivism, which in the progress of knowledge has always seen a guarantee of solving the problems and worries of mankind. And yet, as the poet Zbigniew Herbert says, "the positivists' paradise has proved empty." Though we are entitled to be optimistic, because aren't the achievements of medicine staggering? But then, do they bring us any closer to recognizing the soul? There is not much evidence that they do, for how can we recognize something that we have driven into obscurity, denying it the right to exist? The soul and death: first we displaced the immortal soul from our language and our minds, and now in our thoughts, conversations and daily life we are silencing death. We immerse ourselves in the present. We thrive on it, in the "reality show," the "talk show," and we even take it with us into another life, into a virtual world. In a new Internet phenomenon called "Second Life," an online virtual world that is rapidly attracting millions of users, we do not run about with swords killing monsters. Instead we leave our "reality" for another world, where a virtual home, a virtual car and a virtual spouse await us. In "Second Life" we go to work and earn money. Reuters press agency already has its own permanent correspondent here, and an increasing number of countries have embassies. Here you can make your own face beautiful, shape your figure, style the friends and strangers around you, fall in love and ... spend hours walking about the shops together, buying things for real currency deducted from your credit card. And *Nature*, one of the most prestigious scientific journals, is encouraging scientists to present the results of their latest discoveries at a virtual lecture, in an amphitheater that *Nature* now owns.

♦♦♦

For Heraclitus, the soul posed the trickiest riddle of all. And although he warned that even if we travel all possible roads we shall never reach its limits, he never stopped "looking for himself." In spite of his view that the soul is unattainable, but in accordance with his theory that in a clash of contradictions harmony is born, he kept watching out for the soul in himself. The soul, meaning the essence of the essence. If you look at it like this, you can freely repeat the question about the soul of medicine. You can keep watching out for it, as we have been doing, in the eternal worlds where medicine has always been present — somewhere between life and death, health and illness, science and art, and also in love. In these searches, on our quest, now and then it has twinkled at us in the eyes of a patient awoken from a deep coma, in the transplanted heart of the woman who climbed the Matterhorn, in pain and suffering extinguished by the medical art, or in the glance of a scientist discovering a new medicine. And what if we focus, as in the pupil of an eye, these and other, countless situations into one? Then we will have the encounter between doctor and patient. Along comes the patient with his pain and suffering, his cry for help. And disregarding the patient's fear (and his own), knowing how little he knows (always too little), the doctor says: "I will stand by you. Let us look danger in the face together." And all the doubts our minds have wrapped around the soul for centuries fall away, as a young girl called Kore appears to us in the patient's pupil. There she stands, in bright light, clear as day, in that brief moment when she hears our message: "I will be with you. I will not abandon you. You will not be left alone."

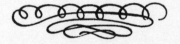

John Martin

AFTERWORD

"Nothing is in the mind that was not previously in the senses," said Aristotle. If we apply that to writing, then the writer creates the work in his mind by processing what has entered through his senses from the outside world. I suppose that is why Wordsworth wrote about daffodils. But Saint John of the Cross wrote about the Dark Night of the Soul. This latter was probably created internally from just a little input via his senses. Whatever is the mix of creativity, the important element is the mixer. For many colleagues in science the mixing would be done by the electrochemistry of the brain, since they believe that there is nothing else than man the molecular machine. But Andrzej Szczeklik was a scientist, and he believed that he had a soul. Whether we can prove that he had a soul is not the important question. Without such a belief all is ultimately futile; with belief in a soul the possibilities of belief in oneself as an infinitely important being at the center of the universe both consciously and unconsciously allow an enhancement of the mixing of the external world and the internal. Even though he read Richard Dawkins's *The Blind Watchmaker* with great interest,

Andrzej believed with conviction that he had a soul and that the world had mystical meaning beyond the molecular.

I remember seeing his Curriculum Vitae once. He listed his interest in music as both "Classic and Romantic." I remember thinking that that summed up Andrzej: the mathematics of Bach and the passion of Chopin. He had spent a year at the Conservatoire in Warsaw studying piano before entering medical school. He would have made a success of either. But perhaps medicine allowed Andrzej to express both classic and romantic tendencies, the kind of thing Bulgakov described in *A Country Doctor's Notebook*.

I remember Andrzej playing Mozart on the grand piano when he stayed in my house in London. But I also remember him playing improvised jazz on an upright piano in a bar in a village in southern Poland.

The pity is that Andrzej died just as he started writing creatively or, alternatively, that he didn't start earlier. He had written hundreds of scientific articles. But that is not writing. It is precise recording that Bach would have understood. Andrzej's romantic writing started only two books before this one. For decades, his time was consumed by the things that he did well: clinical medicine, caring for his patients, science, running a medical school, raising money for research, speaking at conferences. All this kept him from the self that he ultimately found in what we have here called romantic writing. I remember that he wrenched himself away from his unromantic world to spend two weeks alone in his wooden house under the Tatra Mountains to write the first book.

So this book is more than daffodils. It is the product of a soul that has received years of diverse information through the senses and a soul that has matured over the years. The problem for the soul is that its molecular contact with the world is corroding from birth. Thus the dilemma of mature, complex writing: it requires that thing that will end it.

SOURCES

SYMPTOMS AND SHADOWS

3 *To tap and to listen*: Andrzej Szczeklik.

3 *perhaps more than just*: Stanisław Mossakowski, *Program ideowy obrazu Rafa-ela Święta Cecylia* ("The Ideological Plan Behind Raphael's Painting of Saint Cecilia") in *Sztuka jako świadectwo czasu* ("Art as the Testimony of Time"), Warsaw, Arkady, 2005, p. 114.

4 *the immobile face*: Czesław Miłosz, *This*, in *New and Collected Poems 1931–2001*, translated by Czesław Miłosz and Robert Hass, London, Allen Lane, 2001, pp. 663–664.

8 *Duque de Béjar*: J. van Gijn, *The Babinski Sign: A Centenary*, Utrecht, Universiteit Utrecht, 1996, p. 71.

8 *the intervention of our soul*: René Descartes, *Les passions de l'âme*, Paris, Henri le Gras, 1649, quoted in J. van Gijn, op. cit., p. 7.

13 *In both countries*: Seamus Heaney, *In Another Pattern*, lecture given on 12 May 2005 at the Jagiellonian University in Krakow on the occasion of receiving an honorary degree.

13 *when the spirit appearing in nature*: Jarosław Marek Rymkiewicz, *Słowacki. Encyklopedia* ("Słowacki. An Encyclopedia"), Warsaw, Wydawnictwo Sic!, 2004, p. 156.

13 *and further Podolia*: Juliusz Słowacki, *Beniowski*, Canto XI in *Pisma* ("Works"), arranged by A. Górski, Vol. 2, Krakow, Gebethner und Wolff, 1908, p. 479.

14 *Round him a forest of cypress*: Ibid., Canto II, p. 270.

15 *carries in it the seeds of madness*: Gabriel García Márquez, *Tramontana*, in *Strange Pilgrims. Twelve Stories*, translated by Edith Grossman, London, Cape, 1993, p. 135.

15 *drive the sunniest natures*: Nicolas Bouvier, *Journal d'Aran et d'autres lieux*, Paris, Editions Payot, 1990.

ABOUT THE BRAIN

22 *the skull fits the brain*: Ian Glynn, *An Anatomy of Thought. The Origin and Machinery of the Mind*, London, Weidenfeld & Nicolson, 1999, p. 169.

25 *the "notch gene"*: Nick Monk, *Asymmetric Fixation*, "Nature" 2004, Vol. 427, p. 111.

26 *two conscious minds*: Christof Koch, *The Quest for Consciousness. A Neurobiological Approach*, Englewood, Roberts and Co., 2004, p. 294.

29 *long-term, declarative memory*: Greg Miller, *How Are Memories Stored and Retrieved?*, "Science" 2005, Vol. 309, p. 92.

30 *Like an actor*: Christof Koch, *The Quest for Consciousness*, op. cit., p. 196.

30 *epic poem of the night*: Juliusz Kleiner, Włodzimierz Maciąg, *Zarys dziejów literatury polskiej* ("An Outline of the History of Polish Literature"), Wrocław, Zakład Narodowy im. Ossolińskich, 1972, p. 256.

31 Gustavus obiit: Adam Mickiewicz, *Forefathers' Eve*, Part III, in *Polish Romantic Drama: Three Plays in English Translation*, edited by Harold B. Segel, Ithaca, Cornell University Press, 1977, p. 82.

31 *no one can either praise or criticize me*: Sławomir Mrożek, *Baltazar. Autobiografia* ("Baltazar. An Autobiography"), Krakow, Noir sur Blanc, 2006, p. 248.

31 *what makes us whole*: Antoni Libera, introduction to *Baltazar*, Sławomir Mrożek, op. cit., p. 8.

31 *identity split*: Edgardo D. Carosella, Thomas Pradeu, *Transplantation and Identity. A Dangerous Split?*, "The Lancet" 2006, Vol. 368, p. 183.

32 *distance is the essence of beauty*: Czesław Miłosz, *The Land of Ulro*, translated by Louis Iribarne, New York, Farrar, Straus and Giroux, 1985, p. 11.

32 *bountiful memory*: Ibid.

32 *in some material object*: Vladimir Nabokov, *Lectures on Literature*, London, Weidenfeld & Nicolson, 1980, p. 222.

32 *turn years, whole periods*: Czesław Miłosz, *The Land of Ulro*, op. cit., p. 12.

32 *is big screens*: Renata Gorczyńska, *Podróżny świata. Rozmowy z Czesławem Miłoszem* ("World Traveller. Conversations with Czesław Miłosz"), Krakow, Wydawnictwo Literackie, 1992, pp. 139–140.

33 *One need not be a chamber*: Emily Dickinson, "Ghosts," in *Collected Poems of Emily Dickinson*, New York, Avenel Books, 1982, p. 208.

36 *the most striking*: György Buzsáki, *Rhythms of the Brain*, Oxford, Oxford University Press, 2006, p. 370.

37 *Studying and performing music*: Nancy C. Andreasen, *The Creating Brain. The Neuroscience of Genius*, New York, Dana Press, 2005, p. 158.

41 *transmutation of forms*: Andrzej Szczeklik, *Catharsis*, translated by Antonia Lloyd-Jones, Chicago, University of Chicago Press, 2005, p. 24.

43 *What a cruel irony*: Richard Rapport, *Nerve Endings. The Discovery of the Synapse*, New York, W.W. Norton and Co., 2005, p. 184.

43 *Passions are like*: Johann Christian August Heinroth, *Lehrbuch des Seelenge-sundheitskunde* ("Textbook of Mental Health"), Vol. 1, Leipzig, Vogel, 1823, pp. 591–592.

44 *a pitiful city*: Vittorino Andreoli, *I miei mati: Ricordi e storie di un medico della mente* ("My Madmen. Memoirs of a Doctor of the Mind"), Milan, Rizzoli, 2004.

44 *that sleeps all the time*: Edward Shorter, ibid.

44 *For progressive paralysis*: Tadeusz Boy-Żeleński, *Dziadzio* ("Grandpa"), in *Słówka* ("Wordlets"), Warsaw, Książka i Wiedza, 1950, p. 17.

44 *La paralyse générale*: Marie Rivet, *Les aliénés dans la famille et dans la maison de la santé* ("The Insane Within the Family and at the Sanatorium"), Paris, Mason, 1875, p. 145.

46 *in which the patients basked*: Edward Shorter, *A History of Psychiatry. From the Era of the Asylum to the Age of Prozac*, New York, John Wiley & Sons, 1997, p. 147.

46 *was not a true methodology*: Theodore Millon, *Masters of Mind. Exploring the Story of Mental Illness from Ancient Times to the New Millennium*, Hoboken, John Wiley & Sons, 2004, p. 326.

46 *an interruption*: Edward Shorter, *A History of Psychiatry*, op. cit., p. 145.

46 *All sciences have to*: Hans Eysenck, *Decline and Fall of the Freudian Empire*, London, Viking, 1985, p. 207.

48 *wanders astray easily*: Edward Shorter, *A History of Psychiatry*, op. cit., p. 288.

48 *Despite its anchoring*: Edward Shorter, ibid.

48 *walking mines*: Vittorino Andreoli, *I miei mati*, op. cit.

48 *A clear light*: Theodore Millon, *Masters of Mind*, op. cit., p. 588.

IN SEARCH OF THE SOUL

51 *It is only because life is*: Roberto Calasso, *The Marriage of Cadmus and Harmony*, translated by Tim Parks, London, Cape, 1993, p. 117.

51 *Cattle and sheep*: Homer, *The Iliad*, Book IX, verses 406–409, translated by Richmond Lattimore, Chicago, University of Chicago Press, 1951, p. 209.

52 *whenever somebody*: Calasso, *The Marriage* . . . , op. cit., p. 117.

52 *O shining Odysseus*: Homer, *The Odyssey*, Book XI, verses 488–491, translated by Richmond Lattimore, New York, HarperCollins, 1965, p. 180.

52 *On this point*: James George Frazer, *The Belief in Immortality and the Worship of the Dead*, Vol. 1, London, Macmillan, 1913, p. 33.

53 *causing pain, distress and torment*: Jan Parandowski, *Mitologia. Wierzenia i podania Greków i Rzymian* ("Mythology. Beliefs and Tales of the Greeks and Romans"), Warsaw, Czytelnik, 1950, p. 102.

54 *a drop of alien blood*: Erwin Rohde, *Die Religion der Griechen* ("The Religion of the Greeks"), cited in E.R. Dodds, *The Greeks and the Irrational*, Berkeley, University of California Press, 1951, p. 139.

54 *In the seventh century* BC: Dodds, op. cit., p. 140.

55 *Total, agonizing silence*: Wacław Sieroszewski, *Dwanaście lat w kraju Jakutów* ("Twelve Years in the Land of the Yakuts"), Vol. 17, Krakow, Wydawnictwo Literackie, 1961, pp. 327–328, cited in Maria Magdalena Kośko, *Szamanizm. Teatr jednego aktora* ("Shamanism. One-Man Theater"), Poznań, Muzeum Narodowe w Poznaniu, 2002, p. 20.

56 *Orpheus is a Thracian*: Dodds, *The Greeks* . . . , op. cit., p. 147.

The work of the following Poznań-based ethnologists is a rich source of information on the Siberian shamans: Maria Magdalena Kośko, *Mitologia ludów Syberii* ("Mythology of the Peoples of Siberia"), Warsaw, Wydawnictwa Artystyczne i Filmowe, 1990; Kośko, *Szamanism*, op. cit.; Andrzej Rozwadowski and Maria Magdalena Kośko, *Spirits and Stones. Shamanism and Rock Art in Central Asia and Siberia*, Poznań, Instytut Wschodni KAM, 2002; Andrzej Szyjewski, *Szamanizm* ("Shamanism"), Krakow, WAM, 2005.

57 *or at least to lack irreversible time*: Krzysztof Michalski, *The Flame of Eternity. An Interpretation of Nietzsche's Thought*, translated by Benjamin Paloff, Princeton, Princeton University Press, 2012, p. 151.

57 *took hold in European thought*: Ibid., p. 152.

57 *We can compare time*: Arthur Schopenhauer, *The World as Will and Representation*, Vol. 1, translated by E.F.J. Payne, Mineola, New York, Dover, 1969, p. 276, quoted in Michalski, p. 153.

58 *I shall not altogether die*: Horace, Odes III, 30, line 6, *Odes and Epodes*, translated by C.E. Bennett, Cambridge, MA, Harvard University Press, 1952, p. 278–279.

58 *desolate times*: Friedrich Hölderlin, *Bread and Wine*, in *Poems of Holderlin*, translated by Michael Hamburger, London, Nicholson & Watson, 1943, p. 171.

58 *But that which endures*: Friedrich Hölderlin, *Remembrance*, ibid., p. 187.

58 *who knew the secret*: Zbigniew Herbert, *To Ryszard Krynicki. A Letter*, in *The Collected Poems 1956–1998*, translated by Alissa Valles, New York, Ecco, 2007, p. 356.

58 *the value of human life*: John Paul II, *Canonizzazione del Beato Francesco Antonio Fasani* ("Canonization of Blessed Francesco Antonio Fasani"), *Homilies*, 13 April 1986, Vatican, Libreria Editrice Vaticana, 1986.

58 *And if indeed*: Natalya Gorbanevskaya, *Still am Meer* ("[translation of Still am Meer]"), in *Angel dereviannyi* ("Wooden Angel"), Ann Arbor, Ardis, 1982.

58 *in the form of a little doll*: Parandowski, *Mitologia*, op. cit., p. 11.

59 *Kore*: To find the sources and history of the words *kore* and *symbiosis* (which appear in the chapter entitled "Conjunction"), I relied mainly on H.G. Liddell and R. Scott, *A Greek English Lexicon*, Oxford, Oxford University Press, 1996. I was also given invaluable advice and pointers by Professor Stanisław Stabryła, director of the Latin Philology Faculty at the Jagiellonian University, to whom my sincere thanks are due. I also wish to thank Mary R. Lefkowitz, Mellon Professor in the Humanities Emerita, of Wellesley College, Massachusetts.

60 *pounced from the shadows*: Calasso, *The Marriage . . .*, op. cit., p. 210.

60 *drama of the reflection*: Ibid.

61 *do not permit the sight to wander*: Pliny the Elder, *The Natural History*, XI:55, edited and translated by John Bostock and H.T. Riley, London, Taylor & Francis, 1855.

61 *so complete a mirror*: Ibid.

KORE

61 *the eye became*: Calasso, *The Marriage* . . . , op. cit., p. 210.

61 *is to see itself*: Pseudo-Plato, *Alcibiades* 1.133b, 2–3 and 7–10, *Plato in Twelve Volumes*, Vol. 8, translated by W.R.M. Lamb, London, William Heinemann, Ltd., 1955, also available from the Perseus Digital Library, www.perseus.tufts. edu.

61 *Or rather I shall say*: Juliusz Słowacki, *Los mię już żaden nie może zatrwożyć* ("Fate Can Trouble Me No More") in Wacław Borowy, *Od Kochanowskiego do Staffa. Antologia lyriki polskiej* ("An Anthology of Polish Poetry from Kochanowski to Staff"), PIW, Warsaw 1958, p. 258.

62 *O sleep, that teaches*: Jan Kochanowski, *Do snu* ("To Sleep"), translated by Michael J. Mikoś, in *Trifles* on Jan Rybicki's Modern Polish Poetry website, http://www.ap.krakow.pl/nkja/literature/polpoet/kochtrif.htm.

62 *On tankard, plate and sirloin*: Adam Mickiewicz, *Pan Tadeusz*, Book VIII, verses 804–805, translated by Kenneth R. MacKenzie, London, Polish Cultural Foundation, 1986, p. 376.

62 *Take me into your dream*: Ryszard Krynicki, *Weź mnie* ("Take Me") in *Kamień, szron* ("Stone, Rime"), Krakow, Wydawnictwo a5, 2004.

64 Logos, *the invisible spider's thread*: Imre Kertész, *Liquidation*, translated by Tim Wilkinson, New York, Knopf, 2004, p. 97.

64 *Of soul thou shalt never find*: Heraclitus, preserved in Diogenes Laertius, *Lives of Eminent Philosophers*, Book IX, 6–8, translated by R.D. Hicks, Cambridge, MA, Harvard University Press, 1958, Vol. II, p. 415.

64 *the shaman must die*: Mircea Eliade, in Szyjewski, *Szamanizm*, op. cit.

64 *a seasoned expert*: Szyjewski, op. cit., p. 10.

65 *demanded not studying, but exercising*: Władysław Tatarkiewicz, *Historia filozofii* ("A History of Philosophy"), Vol. 1, Warsaw, PWN, 2004, p. 169.

66 *They ask nothing*: Henri Bergson, *The Two Sources of Morality and Religion*, translated by R. Ashley Audra and Cloudsley Brereton, London, Macmillan, 1935, pp. 23–24.

66 *it will never be pure ecstasy*: Pierre Hadot, *Plotinus, or the Simplicity of Vision*, translated by Michael Chase, Chicago, University of Chicago Press, 1993, p. 113.

For more on Plotinus, see Lev Shestov, *In Job's Balance*, translated by Camilla Coventry and C.A. Macartney, London, Dent & Sons, 1932.

66 *Even if this phenomenon*: Hadot, *Plotinus* . . . , op. cit., p. 112.

66 *most vital experience*: Barbara Skarga, *Kwintet Metafizyczny* ("A Metaphysical Quintet"), Krakow, Universitas, 2005, p. 144.

67 *often less pious*: Jean-Noel Vuarnet, *Extases feminines* ("Women's Ecstasies"), Paris, Arthaud, 1980.

68 *a cataplasm of nine leaves*: Jacques Attali, *Blaise Pascal ou le génie français* ("Blaise Pascal or the French genius"), Paris, Fayard, 2000, p. 28.

70 *According to the logic of* cogito, ergo sum: John Paul II, *Memory and Identity: Personal Reflections*, London, Weidenfeld & Nicolson, 2005, pp. 10–11.

71 *weighed as much*: Len Fisher, *Weighing the Soul. The Evolution of Scientific Beliefs*, London, Weidenfeld & Nicolson, 2004, p. 14.

72 *Otherwise, it was*: Szczeklik, *Catharsis*, op. cit., p. 58.

72 *Do not come out into the world*: Saint Augustine, cited in Tatarkiewicz, *Historia filozofii*, op. cit., Vol. 1, p. 195.

72 *a high-ranking officer*: Tomaš Halík, *Co je bez chvění, není pevné. Labyrintem světa a vírou a pochybností* ("If It Doesn't Wobble, It Isn't Certain. The Labyrinth of the World, Faith and Doubt"), Prague, Lidové Noviny, 2002.

72 *except the* coup de grâce: Ibid.

73 *In our earthly house*: Vladimir Nabokov, *The Gift*, translated by D. Nabokov and Michael Scammell with the collaboration of the author, Harmondsworth, Penguin, 1981, p. 283.

73 *to credit marvels*: Seamus Heaney, *Fosterling*, in *Seeing Things*, London, Faber & Faber, 1991, p. 50.

74 *We know — or at least we have been told*: Adam Zagajewski, *The Soul*, translated by Clare Cavanagh, "Agni Magazine," No. 54, Boston University.

75 Christof Koch, *The Quest for Consciousness*, op. cit.

75 Douglas Hofstadter, *I Am a Strange Loop*, New York, Basic Books, 2007.

75 *a mirage, a myth*: Susan Blackmore, *A Strange Sense of Self. Am I a Mirage?*, "Nature" 2007, Vol. 447, p. 29.

75 *which are a light*: H. Nusbaum, lecture, "On the Influence of Spiritual Functions on Matters of Illness," given at the VII Polish Doctors and Naturalists Congress in 1894 in Lwów, quoted in Bartłomiej Dobroczyński, *Idea nieświadomości w polskiej myśli psychologicznej przed Freudem* ("The Idea of the Unconscious Mind in Polish Psychological Thought Before Freud"), Krakow, Universitas, 2005, p. 268.

75 *lack the glow of the conscious mind*: Ibid.

76 *deep epistemological problems*: Colin Blakemore, *In Celebration of Cerebration*, "The Lancet" 2005, Vol. 366, p. 2035.

KORE

77 *consciousness itself cannot have evolved*: Ibid.

77 Antonio Damasio, *The Person Within*, "Nature" 2003, Vol. 423, p. 227.

THE REFLECTED WORLD INSIDE US

81 *continuously ... inhaling*: Sheldon G. Cohen, *Cooke and Vander Veer on Heredity and Sensitization*, "Journal of Allergy and Clinical Immunology" 2002, Vol. 110, p. 674.

81 *I put as much adrenalin*: Ibid., p. 676.

82 *First be a doctor*: Cited in Andrzej Szczeklik, *The Robert Cooke Memorial Lectureship: Aspirin-Induced Asthma*, Annual Meeting of the American Academy of Allergy, Asthma and Immunology, New Orleans 2001.

82 *if he could find a metabolite*: Sheldon G. Cohen, Max Samter, *Excerpts from Classics in Allergy*, Carlsbad, Symposia Foundation, 1992, p. 132.

83 *hair soup*: Jack Howell, *Roger Altounyan and the Discovery of Cromolyn (Sodium Cromoglycate)*, "Journal of Allergy and Clinical Immunology" 2005, Vol. 115, pp. 882–885; Alan M. Edwards, *The Discovery of Cromolyn Sodium and Its Effect on Research and Practice in Allergy and Immunology*, "Journal of Allergy and Clinical Immunology" 2005, Vol. 115, pp. 885–888; and also Alan M. Edwards, Jack Howell, *The Chromones: History, Chemistry and Clinical Development. A Tribute to the Work of Dr. R.E.C. Altounyan*, "Clinical and Experimental Allergy" 2000, Vol. 30, pp. 756–774.

88 *placed in the hands of the physician*: Marvin J. Stone, *Monoclonal Antibodies. Designer Medical Missiles*, "The Lancet" 2006, Vol. 368, pp. S48–S49.

88 *the immune substances*: Paul Ehrlich, quoted in Stone, ibid.

88 *drugs are a delusion*: George Bernard Shaw, *The Doctor's Dilemma*, Act One, London, Constable and Company, Ltd., 1930, p. 24.

93 Quotation from Kierkegaard modified by Jerne, in Thomas Söderqvist, *Science as Autobiography. The Troubled Life of Niels Jerne*, New Haven and London, Yale University Press, 2003, p. 186.

94 *Gradually it has become clear to me*: Friedrich Nietzsche, *Beyond Good and Evil*, translated by Walter Kaufmann, New York, Vintage, 1966, p. 13.

94 *built the edifice*: Tatarkiewicz, *Historia filozofii*, op. cit., Vol. 1, p. 184.

94 *Understand that you are another world*: Juan Eduardo Cirlot, *A Dictionary of Symbols*, translated by Jack Sage, London, Routledge & Kegan Paul, 1962, p. 187.

94 *Perhaps all the dragons*: Rainer Maria Rilke, *Letters to a Young Poet*, translated by Reginald Snell, London, Sidgwick & Jackson, 1945, p. 39.

94 *Perhaps the world was created*: Czesław Miłosz, *Coffer* in *Second Space*, translated by the author and Robert Hass, New York, Ecco, 2004, p. 27.

THE ARCANA OF ART AND THE RIGORS OF SCIENCE

97 *What is truth?*: Mikhail Bulgakov, *The Master and Margarita*, translated by Michael Glenny, London, Harvill, 1988, pp. 33–34.

98 *A correctly uttered magic spell*: Andrzej Szczeklik, *Catharsis*, op. cit., p. 9.

99 Apuleius, *Metamorphoses*, Book XI, 5, in Pierre Hadot, *The Veil of Isis. An Essay on the History of the Idea of Nature*, translated by Michael Chase, Cambridge, Harvard University Press, 2006, p. 236.

100 *the word φύσις*: Ibid., p. 9.

101 *under the torture of experiments*: Francis Bacon, *Novum organum*, quoted in Hadot, *The Veil of Isis*, op. cit., p. 93.

101 *Nature the Sphinx*: Johann W. von Goethe, in Hadot, *The Veil of Isis*, op. cit., p. 249.

101 *One should have more respect*: Friedrich Nietzsche, *The Gay Science*, edited by Bernard Williams, translated by Josefine Nauckhoff and Adrian Del Caro, Cambridge, Cambridge University Press, 2001, p. 8.

101 *Perhaps truth is a woman*: Ibid.

101 *one cannot know anything certain*: Hippocrates, *On Ancient Medicine*, 20, in *The Genuine Works of Hippocrates*, translated by Francis Adams, London, Baillière, Tindall & Cox, 1939, p. 15.

102 *without damage*: Hippocrates, *On Art*, Book XII, 3, in Hadot, *The Veil of Isis*, op. cit., p. 93.

102 In Brueghel's Icarus: W.H. Auden, *Musée des Beaux Arts*, in *W.H. Auden: A Selection By the Poet*, Harmondsworth, Penguin Books, 1958, p. 61.

103 *the phenomenon of the world's indifference*: Leszek Kołakowski, *The Presence of Myth*, translated by Adam Czerniawski, Chicago, University of Chicago Press, 2001, p. 69.

104 *open up spaces for mercy*: John Paul II, *Rise, Let Us Be on Our Way*, London, Jonathan Cape, 2004, p. 75.

110 *we see . . . Galileo's finger*: Peter Atkins, *Galileo's Finger. The Ten Great Ideas of Science*, Oxford, Oxford University Press, 2003, p. 1.

111 *he sat in them himself*: Władysław Szumowski, *Historia medycyny filozoficznie ujęta* ("The History of Medicine Philosophically Expressed"), Sanmedia, 3rd ed., Kraków 1994, p. 477.

111 *universal architecture*: Evelyn Fox Keller, *A Clash of Two Cultures*, "Nature" 2007, Vol. 445, p. 603.

112 *quantum canticle*: Marc Lachieze-Rey and Jean-Pierre Luminet, *Celestial Treasury. From the Music of the Spheres to the Conquest of Space*, Cambridge, Cambridge University Press, 2001, p. 62.

113 *the world was an organism*: Michał Heller, *Filozofia przyrody* ("The Philosophy of Nature"), Krakow, Wydawnictwo Znak, 2004, p. 21.

113 If ever any beauty: John Donne, *The Good-Morrow*, in *Poems of John Donne*, Vol. I, edited by E.K. Chambers, London, Lawrence & Bullen, 1896.

115 *the physics of creative processes*: Michał Heller in *Struktura i emergencja* ("Structure and Emergence"), edited by Michał Heller and Janusz Mączka, Krakow-Tarnów, PAU i Biblos, 2006, p. 33.

115 *by night they devote themselves*: Andrzej Białas, *Wprowadzenie* ("Introduction") in *Struktura i emergencja*, op. cit., p. 33.

116 *There is no such thing as consensus science*: Michael Crichton, "Aliens Cause Global Warming," Caltech Michelin Lecture, 17 January 2003, http://brinnonprosperity.org/crichton2.html.

116 *like a sewer*: Ruth Richardson, *Chance Favours the Prepared Mind*, "The Lancet" 2006, Vol. 368, pp. S46–S47.

116 For the history of the discovery of Hwang's fraud, see "Science" 2006, Vol. 313, p. 22 and "Nature" 2006, Vol. 439, p. 122.

116 On the fraud concerning treatment of cancer of the mouth, see "Nature" 2006, Vol. 439, p. 122.

117 On Jacques Benveniste, see his obituary by Caroline Richmond, *The Guardian*, 21 October 2004.

118 On the controversy between Hooke and Hevelius, see *Naukowa Liga Mistrzów* ("The Scientists' League Championship"), an interview with Lord May of Oxford, "Academia" 2005, No. 3, p. 42.

119 These days success is an idol: Cyprian Kamil Norwid, *Omyłka* ("Mistake") in *Poezja i dobroć. Wybor z utworów* ("Poetry and Goodness. A Selection from His Works"), edited by Marian Piechal, Warsaw, PIW, 1977, p. 658.

119 *Here we have a real*: Andrzej Staruszkiewicz, *Istota sukcesu naukowego* ("The Essence of Scientific Success") in *Sukces w nauce* ("Success in Science"), Warsaw, Fundacja na rzecz Nauki Polskiej, 2006, p. 44.

120 *Vanity is so anchored in the heart of man*: Blaise Pascal, *Pensées*, translated by W.F. Trotter, London, J.M. Dent, 1931, p. 46.

120 The Old Masters: Zbigniew Herbert, *Old Masters*, in *The Collected Poems*, op. cit., p. 345.

121 *the principle of limited sloppiness*: *Inspiring Science. Jim Watson and the Age of DNA*, edited by John R. Inglis, Joseph Sambrook and Jan A. Witkowski, New York, Cold Spring Harbor Laboratory Press, 2003, p. 126.

125 *conception of Nature*: Robert J. Richards, *The Romantic Conception of Life. Science and Philosophy in the Age of Goethe*, Chicago, University of Chicago Press, 2002, p. 516; and also Manfred D. Laublicher, *A Premodern Synthesis*, "Science" 2003, Vol. 299.

126 *I am at present fit only to read Humboldt*: Charles Darwin, *Beagle Diary*, quoted in Richards, op. cit., p. 514.

126 *I never forget*: Charles Darwin, in a letter to Joseph Hooker dated 10 February 1845, quoted in Richards, op. cit., p. 514.

126 *You have without perceiving it*: Letter from Caroline Darwin to Charles Darwin dated 28 October 1833, quoted in Richards, op. cit., p. 521.

126 *organic crystallography*: Olaf Breidbach, *Visions of Nature. The Art and Science of Ernst Haeckel*, New York, Prestel, 2006, p. 105.

127 *Their very beauty betrays them*: Philip Ball, *Painting the Whole Picture?*, "Nature" 2007, Vol. 445, p. 486.

127 *life navigates to precise end-points*: Simon Conway Morris, *Life's Solution. Inevitable Humans in a Lonely Universe*, Cambridge and New York, Cambridge University Press, 2003, Preface, p. xiii.

128 *the best example of convergent evolution in human beings*: Erika Check, *How Africa Learned to Love a Cow*, "Nature" 2006, Vol. 444, pp. 994–996.

GENETICS AND CANCER

131 *an apparent end*: Franz Kafka, *Diaries*, quoted in Guido Ceronetti, *The Silence of the Body: Materials for the Study of Medicine*, translated by Michael Moore, New York, Farrar, Straus and Giroux, 1993, p. 203.

131 *souls are all exempt from power of death*: Ovid, *Metamorphoses*, translated by Brookes More, Boston, Cornhill Publishing Co., 1922, Book 15, line 158.

131 I am the family face: Thomas Hardy, *Heredity*, in *The Complete Poems of Thomas Hardy*, edited by James Gibson, London, Macmillan, 1976, p. 434.

132 *gemmules*: Charles Darwin, *The Variation of Plants and Animals Under Domestication*, London, John Murray, 1868, quoted in Tim Lewens, *Science Undermined by Our Limited Imagination?*, "Science" 2006, Vol. 313, p. 1047.

133 *we will know what it is to be human*: W. Gilbert, cited in Richard Lewontin, *The Triple Helix*, Cambridge, Harvard University Press, 2001, p. 11.

133 *We have the sequence now*: J. Michael Bishop, *How to Win the Nobel Prize*, Cambridge, Harvard University Press, 2003, p. 217.

133 *The fact that the genome was "decoded"*: See D.A. Wheeler et al., *The Complete Genome of an Individual by Massively Parallel DNA Sequencing*, "Nature" 2008, Vol. 452, p. 877.

134 *on what Watson wrote*: M.V. Olson, *Dr. Watson's Base Pair*, "Nature" 2008, Vol. 452, p. 819.

134 *"personalized" colors*: See F.R. Collins, *The Language of Life. DNA and the Revolution in Personalised Medicine*, London, Profile Books, 2010.

135 *an individual's risk*: Ibid., p. 90.

135 *an all-inclusive price*: L.J. Kricka et al., *Ethics Watch. Direct Access Genetic Testing. The View from Europe*, "Nature Reviews, Genetics" 2011, Vol. 12, p. 670.

136 *the clinical repercussions of the discovery*: See H. Varmus, *Ten Years On. The Human Genome and Medicine*, "New England Medicine" 2010, Vol. 362, pp. 2028–9.

137 *(non-baryonic) matter that is different from ours*: Stanisław Bajtlik, *The Beginning of the Universe*, "Academia" 2004, No. 1, pp. 5–7.

137 *black*: *The Dark Side*, "Science" (special edition) 2003, Vol. 300, p. 1893.

137 *junk*: Christian Biémont, Cristina Vieira, *Junk DNA as an Evolutionary Force*, "Nature" 2006, Vol. 443, p. 521.

137 *nature's evolutionary experiments*: Wojciech Makałowski, *Not Junk After All*, "Science" 2003, Vol. 300, p. 1246.

140 On the new definition of a gene, see Helen Pearson, *What Is a Gene?*, "Nature" 2006, Vol. 441, p. 398.

144 For more on Hermann Joseph Muller, see Elof Axel Carlson, *Genes, Radiation and Society. The Life and Work of H.J. Muller*, Ithaca, Cornell University Press, 1981, p. 174.

144 *my period of usefulness*: J. Michael Bishop, *How to Win a Nobel Prize*, op. cit., p. 150.

SOURCES

144 *And finally*: Theodor Boveri, *The Origin of Malignant Tumors*, Baltimore, Williams and Wilkins, 1929, pp. 26–27.

145 *landmark conclusions*: J. Michael Bishop, *How to Win a Nobel Prize*, op. cit., p. 152.

145 *22,910 somatically acquired substitutions*: E.D. Pleasance et al., *A Small-Cell Lung Cancer Genome with Complex Signatures of Tobacco Exposure*, "Nature" 2010, Vol. 463, p. 184.

145 *this number totaled 33,345*: E.D. Pleasance et al., *A Comprehensive Catalogue of Somatic Mutations from a Human Cancer Genome*, "Nature" 2010, Vol. 463, p. 191.

147 *In experience, understood as*: Bogusław Maciejewski, in *Dobry zawód. Z lekarzami rozmawiają Krystyna Bochenek i Dariusz Kortko* ("A Good Profession. Conversations with Doctors by Krystyna Bochenek and Dariusz Kortko"), Krakow, Wydawnictwo Znak, 2006, p. 305.

149 *five hundred and eighteen genes*: See Christopher Greenman et al., *Patterns of Somatic Mutation in Human Cancer Genomes*, "Nature" 2007, Vol. 446, p. 153.

149 *drivers . . . passengers*: See Daniel A. Haber, Jeff Settleman, *Drivers and Passengers*, "Nature" 2007, Vol. 446, p. 145.

THE TRUTHS OF BIOLOGY AND FAITH

151 *There are two popular myths about Charles Darwin*: John Gribbin, *The Scientists*, New York, Random House, 2002, p. 339.

151 *the most important event of my life*: Charles Darwin, quoted in Niles Eldredge, *Darwin. Discovering the Tree of Life*, New York, W.W. Norton & Co., 2005, p. 14.

152 *I always feel as if*: John Gribbin, *The Scientists*, op. cit., p. 346.

153 *literally made plants sexy*: Ibid., p. 332.

154 *like confessing a murder*: Charles Darwin, quoted in Niles Eldredge, *Darwin*, op. cit., p. 43.

156 omnis cellula e cellula: Rudolf Virchow's famous sentence.

156 *Nothing in biology makes sense*: Theodosius Dobzhansky, cited in Niles Eldredge, *Darwin*, op. cit., p. 16.

156 *essentially a historical theory*: Paul Nurse, *The Great Ideas of Biology*, "Clinical Medicine" 2003, Vol. 3, pp. 560–568.

158 *symbiogenesis*: Lynn Margulis, *Symbiotic Theory of the Origin of Eukaryotic Organelles*, in *Symbiosis Symposium 29 of the Society for Experimental Biology*, edited by D.L. Lee and D.H. Jennings, Cambridge, Cambridge University Press, 1975, pp. 21–38; and Lynn Margulis and Dorion Sagan, *Acquiring Genomes. A Theory of the Origins of Species*, New York, Basic Books, 2002.

158 *one of the greatest enigmas*: James A. Lake, *Disappearing Act*, "Nature" 2007, Vol. 446, p. 983.

158 *one of the most mysterious questions*: Christian de Duve, *The Origin of Eukaryotes. A Reappraisal*, "Nature Reviews, Genetics" 2007, Vol. 8, p. 395.

158 *is not due to random events*: Axel Mayer, *Viewing Life as a Cooperation. Can Symbiosis and Genome Acquisition Account for All Speciation?*, "Nature" 2002, Vol. 418, p. 275.

159 *albeit with some novelties*: Sean Nee, *The Great Chain of Being*, "Nature" 2005, Vol. 435, p. 429.

160 *the Indo-European languages*: See William Jones in Robert Claiborne, *The Life and Times of the English Language*, London, Bloomsbury, 1990, p. 22.

160 *The resemblance between German and Dutch*: Richard Dawkins, *The Ancestor's Tale*, Boston, Houghton Mifflin, 2004, p. 25.

160 *ring of life*: Maria C. Rivera, James A. Lake, *The Ring of Life Provides Evidence for a Genome Fusion Origin of Eukaryotes*, "Nature" 2004, Vol. 431, p. 152.

161 *more than DNA*: Elizabeth Culotta, *What Genetic Changes Made Us Uniquely Human*, "Science" 2005, Vol. 309, p. 91.

161 *Thus, from the genomic perspective*: Svante Pääbo, *The Mosaic That Is Our Genome*, "Nature" 2003, Vol. 421, p. 409.

161 On the Neanderthal genome, see Richard E. Green et al., *Analysis of One Million Base Pairs of Neanderthal DNA*, "Nature" 2006, Vol. 444. p. 330.

162 *We are survival machines*: Cited in Dan Sperber, *Evolution of the Selfish Gene*, "Nature" 2006, Vol. 441, p. 151.

162 The Selfish Gene *has been, and remains*: Ibid.

163 *Many of the fundamental questions about evolution*: Tom Kirkwood, *Thank God for Richard Dawkins?*, "The Lancet" 2006, Vol. 368, p. 1955.

163 *a special difficulty*: Charles Darwin, cited in Oliver Curry, *One Good Deed. Can a Simple Equation Explain the Development of Altruism?*, "Nature" 2006, Vol. 444, p. 683.

164 *costly acts*: Ernst Fehr, Urs Fischbacher, *The Nature of Human Altruism*, "Nature" 2003, Vol. 425, p. 785.

164 *posterior superior temporal cortex*: Dharol Tankersley, C. Jill Stowe, Scott A. Huettel, *Altruism Is Associated with an Increased Neural Response to Agency*, "Nature Neuroscience" 2007, Vol. 10, pp. 150–151.

164 *Current gene-based evolutionary theories*: Ernst Fehr, Urs Fischbacher, *The Nature of Human Altruism*, op. cit., p. 785.

164 *Fifty-four percent of U.S. adults*: David Sloan Wilson, *Evolution for Everyone. How Darwin's Theory Can Change the Way We Think About Our Lives*, New York, Delacorte Press, 2007, p. 2.

165 *Darwin made it possible*: Richard Dawkins, *The Blind Watchmaker. Why the Evidence of Evolution Reveals a Universe Without Design*, New York, Norton, 1986, cited in Michael Shermer, *The Blind Godmaker*, "Science" 2005, Vol. 308, pp. 205–206.

165 *I'm a Darwinist*: Richard Dawkins in *The Third Culture*, edited by John Brockman, New York, Simon and Schuster, 1995, pp. 75–95, cited in Michael Shermer, *The Blind Godmaker*, op. cit.

165 *The universe we observe*: Richard Dawkins, *River Out of Eden. A Darwinian View of Life*, London, Weidenfeld and Nicholson, 1995, cited in Michael Shermer, *The Blind Godmaker*, op. cit.

166 Have we really lost faith in that other space?: Czesław Miłosz, *Second Space*, op. cit., p. 3.

166 *in our serfdom, in our defenselessness*: Renata Gorczyńska, *Podróżny świata* ("World Traveller"), op. cit., 139.

166 Richard Dawkins, *The God Delusion*, London, Bantam Press, 2006. Polemic with Dawkins's theses aiming to speak in favor of the non-existence of God has been undertaken by Alister E. McGrath and Joanna Collicutt McGrath in *The Dawkins Delusion*, London, SPCK, 2007.

166 *so easily in opposition*: Tom Kirkwood, *Thank God for Richard Dawkins?*, op. cit., p. 1955.

167 *Darwinian fundamentalist*: This was how Stephen Jay Gould described Richard Dawkins, cited in Michael Shermer, *The Blind Godmaker*, op. cit.

167 Francis S. Collins, *The Language of God*, New York, Free Press, 2006.

167 *makes man His confidant*: Józef Życiński, *Bóg i ewolucja* ("God and Evolution"), Lublin, TN KUL, 2002, p. 197.

KORE

167 *anti-scientific*: Erika Check, *Genomics Luminary Weighs In on U.S. Faith Debate*, "Nature" 2006, Vol. 442, p. 114.

168 *What does Athens have in common with Jerusalem?*: Tertullian, *De praescriptione haereticorum*, Book VII, 9: *"Quid ergo Athenis et Hierosolymis? Quid academiae et ecclesiae?,"* cited in John Paul II, *Fides et Ratio* ("Faith and Reason") (Encyclicals), Vatican, Libreria Editrice Vaticana 1998, Chapter IV, 41.

168 *meaning ... comes only from the* sacrum: Leszek Kołakowski, cited in Father Józef Sadzik, *Inne niebo, inna ziemia* ("Another Heaven, Another Earth"), introduction to the Polish edition of *The Land of Ulro* by Czesław Miłosz, *Ziemi Ulro*, Krakow, Wydawnictwo Znak, 2000.

168 *Faith and reason* (fides et ratio) *are like two wings* ... : John Paul II, *Fides et Ratio*, op. cit.

THE BORDERLANDS

172 *particle ... cell*: Steven Salzberg et al., *Journal Club*, "Nature" 2005, Vol. 438, p. 133.

172 *mimivirus*: D. Raoult et al., *The 1.2-Megabase Genome Sequence of Mimivirus*, "Science" 2004, Vol. 306, p. 1344.

175 *usually had numerous other infections*: Roberto C. Gallo, Luc Montagnier, *The Discovery of HIV as the Cause of AIDS*, "The New England Journal of Medicine" 2003, Vol. 349, p. 2283.

177 *Only one fifth of people*: Kent A. Sepkowitz, *One Disease, Two Epidemics. AIDS at 25*, "The New England Journal of Medicine" 2006, Vol. 354, p. 2411.

178 *hepatitis developed in*: J. Garrott Allen et al., *Blood Transfusions and Serum Hepatitis*, "Annals of Surgery" 1959, Vol. 150, p. 455.

179 *The benefits were instantaneous*: Jacalyn Duffin, *Lovers and Livers. Disease Concepts in History*, Toronto, University of Toronto Press, 2005, p. 92.

182 *theory of cyclooxygenase aspirin-induced asthma*: Andrzej Szczeklik, Ryszard Gryglewski, Grażyna Czerniawska-Mysik, *Relationship of Inhibition of Prostaglandin Biosynthesis by Analgesics to Asthma Attacks in Aspirin-Sensitive Patients*, "British Medical Journal" 1975, Vol. 1, pp. 67–69; and Andrzej Szczeklik, Donald D. Stevenson, *Aspirin-Induced Asthma: Advances in Pathogenesis, Diagnosis and Management*, "Journal of Allergy and Clinical Immunology" 2003, Vol. 111, pp. 913–921.

185 *the number of cells produced*: J. Michael Bishop, *How to Win the Nobel Prize*, op. cit., p. 143.

SOURCES

186 *it was the virus that invented DNA*: Patrick Forterre, *The Two Ages of the RNA World, and the Transition to the DNA World. A Story of Viruses and Cells*, "Biochimie" 2005, Vol. 87, pp. 793–803.

186 *the RNA world*: John Withfield, *Base Invaders*, "Nature" 2006, Vol. 439, p. 130.

188 *the rough, ropelike tail*: Robert M. Hazen, *Genesis. The Scientific Quest for Life's Origin*, Washington, D.C., Joseph Henry Press, 2005, p. xvii.

188 *an agreed-upon definition of the term life*: Gerald Joyce, *Foreword*, in *Origins of Life. The Central Concepts*, edited by David W. Deamer, Gail R. Fleischaker, Boston, Jones and Bartlett, 1994, pp. xi–xii.

189 *the oldest, primordial bacteria … the Loch Ness monster*: The famous controversy of 2002 between William Schopf, the discoverer of life at the oldest excavations dating back more than 3.7 billion years, and Martin William Brasier, who denied the accuracy of these discoveries, was described in a book by Andrew H. Knoll, *Life on a Young Planet. The First Three Billion Years of Evolution on Earth*, Princeton, Princeton University Press, 2003, pp. 60–65.

190 *a number of pieces were collected*: Robert M. Hazen, *Genesis*, op. cit., p. 69.

190 *a primitive Earth*: Ibid., p. 87.

191 *primordial or prebiotic soup*: The soup metaphor was introduced by J.B.S. Haldane in *The Origin of Life*, "The Rationalist Annual" 1929, pp. 3–10.

192 Günter Wächtershäuser, *Life As We Don't Know It*, "Science" 2000, Vol. 289, p. 1307.

192 Albert Eschenmoser, *Chemical Etiology of Nucleic Acid Structure*, "Science" 1999, Vol. 284, p. 2118; and *The TNA-Family of Nucleic Acid Systems: Properties and Prospects*, "Origins of Life and Evolution of Biosphere" 2004, Vol. 34, p. 277.

192 *could be that quantum mechanics*: Paul Davies, *A Quantum Recipe for Life*, "Nature" 2005, Vol. 437, p. 819.

193 *attempts to define life*: Carol Cleland, Christopher Chyba, quoted in Robert M. Hazen, *Genesis*, op. cit., p. 30.

ON DYING AND DEATH

195 *But there are a thousand ways to die*: Ovid, *Heroides*, Book X, p. 81.

196 An immense coldness: Zbigniew Herbert, *The Longobards*, in *Selected Poems*, translated by Czesław Miłosz and Peter Dale Scott, Manchester, Carcanet, 1985, p. 127.

198   *life involves maturing*: Ewa Błaszczyk, Krystyna Strączek, *Wejść tam nie można* ("You Cannot Go In There"), Krakow, Wydawnictwo Znak, 2005.

198   *playing a game of tennis ... visiting all the rooms of her house*: Adrian M. Owen et al., *Detecting Awareness in the Vegetative State*, "Science" 2006, Vol. 313, p. 1402.

199   *necessary or sufficient*: Paul Matthews, quoted in Michael Hopkin, *Vegetative Patient Shows Signs of Conscious Thought*, "Nature" 2006, Vol. 443, p. 132.

199   *neurons in his brain*: Hopkin, ibid., p. 133. For the original contribution, see Henning U. Voss et al., *Possible Axonal Regrowth in Late Recovering from the Minimally Conscious State*, "The Journal of Clinical Investigation" 2006, Vol. 116, p. 2005.

200   *If the sick or dying person*: Tadeusz Biesaga, *Kontrowersje wokół nowej definicji śmierci* ("Controversies Around the New Definition of Death"), "Medycyna Praktyczna" 2006, No. 2, pp. 20–23.

201   *But in spite of that the decision was taken*: Tomasz Trojanowski, *Człowiek umiera dwa razy* ("A Person Dies Twice"), *Rzeczpospolita*, 22–23 October 2005, "Plus Minus" supplement, p. 8.

202   *desperate longing for grace*: Helen Langdon, *Caravaggio: A Life*, London, Chatto & Windus, 1998, p. 372.

202   *It is not necessary*: Francesco Susinno, quoted in Howard Hibbard, *Caravaggio*, New York, Harper & Row, 1983, p. 386.

203   *resurrectionists*: Mary Roach, *Stiff*, London, Penguin Books, 2004, p. 43.

204   *I think your solution*: John J. Ross, reviewing *The Knife Man. The Extraordinary Life and Times of John Hunter, Father of Modern Surgery* by Wendy Moore, in "The New England Journal of Medicine" 2005, Vol. 353, p. 2412.

204   *An armed savage*: Ibid.

205   *see what's under your hood*: Donald Jenkins, quoted in John Bohannon, *Anatomy's Full Monty*, "Science" 2003, Vol. 301, pp. 1172–1175.

205   *the Walt Disney of Death*: Ibid. See also Penny Herscovitch, *Rest in Plastic*, "Science" 2003, Vol. 299, p. 828.

206   *one major idea dominates*: Chantal Delsol, *The Unlearned Lessons of the Twentieth Century: An Essay on Late Modernity*, translated by Robin Dick, Wilmington, Delaware, ISI Books, 2006, p. 32.

207   *encourage a person to be pious*: Ignacy Chrzanowski, *Historia literatury niepodległej Polski* ("A History of the Literature of Independent Poland"), Warsaw, PIW, 1974, p. 59.

208 *Every doctor's a cheating fraud*: Ibid., p. 61.

209 *the rattle of bones*: Jacques Le Goff, Nicolas Truong, *Une histoire du corps au Moyen Âge*, Paris, Liana Levi, 2003, p. 139.

209 *the dance of the spindleshanks*: Ibid.

209 *a waiting room for ordinary sinners*: Jacques Le Goff, *The Birth of Purgatory*, translated by Arthur Goldhammer, Chicago, University of Chicago Press, 1984.

209 *Death is a scandal, just like pain and suffering*: Bronisław Wildstein, *Godność umierania i ludzkiego życia* ("The Dignity of Dying and Human Life"), *Rzeczpospolita*, 27 August 2004, p. A7.

209 *The contrast between suffering and joy*: Johan Huizinga, *The Waning of the Middle Ages*, translated by F. Hopman, Harmondsworth, Penguin Books, 1985, p. 9.

210 *We would recall*: Benedetto Croce, *The Conduct of Life*, translated by Arthur Livingston, London, Harrap, 1925, p. 35.

210 *in all these strivings*: Ibid., p. 36.

211 *'Death is a master from Germany'*: Joanna Roszak, *Wystawa "Taniec śmierci"* ("'Dance of Death' Exhibition"), "Zeszyty Literackie" 2003, No. 2, p. 141.

211 *painted with tangible precision*: Kazimierz Wyka, *Thanatos i Polska, czyli o Jacku Malczewskim* ("Thanatos and Poland, or On Jacek Malczewski"), Krakow, Wydawnictwo Literackie, 1971, p. 48.

211 *She is young—so she has time to wait ...* : Andrzej Wajda, *O śmierci na obrazach Jacka Malczewskiego* ("On Death in Jacek Malczewski's Paintings"), "Medycyna Praktyczna" 2003, No. 1, p. 16.

212 *unity with whatever man*: Adam Heydel, *Jacek Malczewski*, Krakow, Wydawnictwo Literacko-Naukowe, 1933, p. 229.

212 *the clocks began to turn*: Adam Zagajewski, *Życie nie jest snem* ("Life Is Not a Dream") translated by Clare Cavanagh, in *Eternal Enemies*, New York, Farrar. Straus and Giroux, 2008, p. 107.

212 *the whole thing must oxidise ... should change the enterprise*: Jacek Dehnel, *Il Sogno*, translated by George Szirtes.

213 *She is a body in your body*: Marzanna Kielar, *Death Has Furnished Her Lair Inside You*, in *Salt Monody*, translated by Elżbieta Wójcik-Leese, Boston, Zephyr Press, 2006, p. 103.

213 *we find it, like something*: Sándor Márai, Diaries.

213 *second childishness*: William Shakespeare, *As You Like It*, Act II, scene 7.

214 *he had come home to himself*: Seamus Heaney, *The Door Stands Open*: *Czesław Miłosz, 1911–2004*, Dublin, Irish Writer's Centre, 2005.

214 *it does not have to be nothing but decay*: Sándor Márai, Diaries.

215 "My children," he said: Seamus Heaney, "What Passed at Colonus" in *The Door Stands Open*, op. cit.

215 *like grains of sand pouring through a sieve*: Giuseppe Tomasi di Lampedusa, quoted in Sándor Márai, Diaries.

216 *Everyone unanimously admits*: Władysław Tatarkiewicz, *Historia filozofii*, Vol. 1, op. cit., p. 73.

216 *Crito, we ought to offer a cock*: Plato, *Phaedo*, 117, translated by Hugh Tredennick, Harmondsworth, Penguin Books, 1975, p. 183.

216 *Socrates wanted to die*: Friedrich Nietzsche, *Twilight of the Idols*, in *The Portable Nietzsche*, translated by W. Kaufmann, New York, Viking Books, 1973, p. 479.

216 *To die proudly*: Ibid., p. 536.

216 *death at the right time*: Ibid.

217 *Maybe it will be in this position*: Jarosław Marek Rymkiewicz, *Słowacki*, op. cit., p. 338.

217 *worked some more on the phrase*: Ibid., p. 339.

217 *the time has come to cast off*: Ibid.

217 *suddenly amid the group*: Giuseppe Tomasi di Lampedusa, *The Leopard*, translated by Archibald Colquhoun, Everyman's Library, 1991, p. 193.

217 *It is a matter of prime importance*: J. Mersen, in a letter to Andrzej Szczeklik, 15 December 2005.

218 *But a common night awaiteth every man: Sed omnes una manet nox / et calcanda semel via leti*, Horace, op. cit., *Odes*, Book I, 28, ll. 15–16, p. 77.

218 *essential for closing the most important stage*: Jacek Łuczak and Marzena Studniarek, *Przygotowanie do umierania i śmierci* ("Preparing for Dying and Death") in *Choroby wewnętrzne* ("Internal Diseases"), edited by Andrzej Szczeklik, Vol. 2, Krakow, Medycyna Praktyczna, 2006, p. 2310.

219 *the metaphysical isolation*: Father Zbigniew Pawlak, *Aspekty duchowe opieki paliatywnej* ("Spiritual Aspects of Palliative Care") in *Choroby wewnętrzne*, Vol. 2, op. cit., p. 2307.

219 *One should not fear silence*: Ibid., p. 2308.

220 *Some people thought*: Stanisław Lem, *Rwąca fala* ("Rushing Wave") in *Czu-wanie, 1–8 kwietnia 2005* ("The Vigil, 1–8 April 2005"), Krakow, Wydawnictwo Znak, 2005, p. 123.

221 *Anyone who witnessed the passing*: Father Adam Boniecki, *Jan Paweł II. Papież na trudne czasy* ("John Paul II. A Pope for Difficult Times") in *Czu-wanie*, op. cit., p. 232.

PROMETHEAN AMBITIONS

225 For details of treating lower limb ischemia with stem cell transplantation, see Rafał Niżankowski et al., *The Treatment of Advanced Chronic Lower Limb Ischaemia with Marrow Stem Cell Autotransplantation*, "Kardiologia Polska" 2005, Vol. 63, pp. 351–360.

226 *I shall cite an unusual example*: See P. Macchiarini et al., *Clinical Trans-plantation of a Tissue-Engineered Airway*, "The Lancet" 2008, Vol. 372, p. 2023–2030.

227 *Mixed cells give mixed results*: Anthony Rosenzweig, *Cardiac Cell Therapy. Mixed Results from Mixed Cells*, "The New England Journal of Medicine" 2006, Vol. 355, p. 1274.

228 *we should still be surprised*: Ian Wilmut, quoted in Erika Check, *Dolly. A Hard Act to Follow*, "Nature" 2007, p. 445, p. 802.

228 *Cloning is still essentially a black box*: Robert Lanza, quoted in Erika Check, *Dolly. A Hard Act to Follow*, op. cit.

229 The breakthrough discovery about reprogramming mature cells is described by Kazutoshi Takahashi et al., *Induction of Pluripotent Stem Cells from Adult Human Fibroblasts by Defined Factors*, "Cell" 2007, Vol. 131, p. 861; Junying Yu et al., *Induced Pluripotent Stem Cell Lines Derived from Human Somatic Cells*, "Science" 2007, Vol. 318, p. 1917; In-Hyun Park et al., *Reprogramming of Human Somatic Cells to Pluripotency with Defined Factors*, "Nature" 2008, Vol. 451, p. 141.

230 *People working on ethics*: Gretchen Kogel and Constance Holden, *Field Leaps Forward with New Stem Cell Advances*, "Science" 2007, Vol. 318, p. 1225.

230 *the road to clinical application*: See E. Dolgin, *Flaw in Induced-Stem-Cell Model*, "Nature" 2011, Vol. 470, p. 13.

230 *genetic and epigenetic abnormalities*: M.F. Pera, *Stem Cells: The Dark Side of Induced Pluripotency*, "Nature" 2011, Vol. 471, p. 46.

230 *In music, the linear passage of time*: See K. Berger, *Bach's Cycle, Mozart's Arrow*, Berkeley and Los Angeles, University of California Press, 2007.

KORE

232 *To make a Toad or Serpent*: John Locke, quoted in William R. Newman, *Promethean Ambitions. Alchemy and the Quest to Perfect Nature*, Chicago, University of Chicago Press, 2004, p. 164.

236 *to move in all dimensions and directions*: Ibid., p. 297.

236 *tendency to the beautiful*: Ibid., p. 298.

236 *a symbol for the human intellect*: Ibid.

238 Nature did well: *Dante's Inferno*, Canto XXXI, verses 49–54, translated by J.G. Nichols, London, Hesperus Poetry, 2005, p. 323.

242 *keep the mythical blood in circulation*: Roberto Calasso, *The Marriage of Cadmus and Harmony*, op. cit., p. 281.

242 *like faint apparitions out of dreams*: Jan Parandowski, *Mitologia. Wierzenia i podania Greków i Rzymian* ("Mythology. The Beliefs and Tales of the Greeks and Romans"), London, Wydawnictwo Puls, 1992, p. 45.

243 You think you freed him?: Ted Hughes, *Alcestis*, London, Faber & Faber, 2000, p. 58.

243 *between good and evil*: Barbara Skarga, *Ślad i obecność* ("Trace and Presence"), Warsaw, PWN, 2002, p. 188.

244 *a model of life that is not conditioned by norms*: Janusz Sławiński, *Postmodernizm* ("Postmodernism") in *Słownik terminów literackich* ("A Dictionary of Literary Terms") edited by Michał Głowiński et al., Wrocław, Zakład Narodowy im. Ossolińskich, 2002, pp. 412–415.

244 *is established without our involvement*: See Abraham Joshua Heschel, *Man Is Not Alone. A Philosophy of Religion*, New York, Farrar, Straus and Young, 1951.

THE ENCHANTMENT OF LOVE

247 Some say that the most beautiful thing: Sappho, quoted in Oliver Taplin, *Greek Fire*, London, Jonathan Cape, 1989, p. 141.

248 *the passion of those who are incessantly preoccupied*: Oribasius of Pergamon, quoted in Jacalyn Duffin, *Lovers and Livers*, op. cit., p. 49.

248 *The patients should be submerged*: Le Menuet, in *Memoires de l'Academie Royale des Sciences. Histoire*, 1734, p. 56.

249 *the beloved is described as*: Jacalyn Duffin, *Lovers and Livers*, op. cit., p. 43.

249 J.D.T. Bienville, *De la nymphomanie*, Amsterdam, 1778, pp. 171–172, quoted in Michel Foucault, *The History of Madness*, translated by Jonathan Murphy and Jean Khalfa, London, Routledge, 2006, p. 322.

249 *they were sometimes that too*: Robert Calasso, *Literature and the Gods*, translated by Tim Parks, London, Vintage, 2001, p. 30.

250 *the recomposition is enacted*: Michel Foucault, *The History of Madness*, op. cit., p. 324.

251 she envisioned between: Joseph Brodsky, *Aeneas and Dido*, translated by Zara M. Torlone, http://nauplion.net/DIDO.html.

251 Tongue of adder: Władysław Kopaliński, *Słownik mitów i tradycji kultury* ("A Dictionary of the Myths and Traditions of Culture"), Warsaw, PIW, 1985, p. 612.

252 *at once a source of joy and pain*: Maria Immacolata Macioti, *Miti e magie delle erbe*, Rome, Newton Compton Editori, 1993.

252 *the erotic act*: Krzysztof Michalski, *The Flame of Eternity*, op. cit., p. 136.

253 *blameless culprits, sinless sinners*: Wisława Szymborska, *Posłowie* ("Afterword") in Joseph Bedier, *The Romance of Tristan and Iseult*, in Polish translation as *Dzieje Tristana i Izoldy*, translated by Tadeusz Boy-Żeleński, Krakow, Wydawnictwo Literackie, 1996, p. 142.

253 *we should forgive them*: Ibid.

253 *born not from life*: Ibid.

255 *music is a secret arithmetical exercise*: Gottfried Wilhelm von Leibniz.

256 *he had been filled with love*: Marcel Proust, *In Search of Lost Time*, Vol. 1, *Swann's Way*, translated by C.K. Scott Moncrieff and Terence Kilmartin, London, Chatto & Windus, 1992, p. 251.

256 *love is all there is*: Emily Dickinson, *That Love Is All There Is*, Poem 1765 in *The Complete Poems of Emily Dickinson*, edited by Thomas H. Johnson, London, Faber & Faber, 1875, p. 714.

256 *for her, loneliness begins*: Jean Giraudoux, *Ondine*, Act I, Scene 9, Paris, Edition Grasset, 1990, p. 49.

257 *He who breaks his sacred vow; Rumor has it that Ondines appear*: Adam Mickiewicz, *Świtezianka*, in *Dzieła* ("Works"), Vol. 1, *Ballady i romanse* ("Ballads and Romances"), Warsaw, Czytelnik, 1949, p. 19.

259 J.M. Coetzee, *Slow Man*, New York, Viking, 2005.

259 *whose sex appeal relies*: Magdalena Miecznicka, *Coetzee tęskni za miłością* ("Coetzee Longs for Love"), "Dziennik," 28–29 October 2006, p. 31.

260 *yes, in spite of all*: John Keats, *Endymion: A Poetic Romance*, Book I, verses 11–13, *Keats' Poetical Works*, London, Oxford University Press, 1944, p. 57.

260 *That little shiver*: Vladimir Nabokov, *Lectures on Literature*, op. cit., p. 64.

261 *If we are not capable*: Ibid.

261 *although ... surely deep in our hearts*: Adam Zagajewski in a letter to Andrzej Szczeklik, 15 November 2003.

261 *in which the blood of mystery circulates*: Bruno Schulz, in a letter to Stanisław Ignacy Witkiewicz dated 1935, quoted in Bruno Schulz, *Księga listów* ("Big Book of Letters"), edited by Jerzy Ficowski, Gdańsk, słowo/obraz terytoria, 2002, p. 100.

261 *to reach a single, empirical answer*: Adam Zagajewski in a letter to Andrzej Szczeklik, 15 November 2003.

262 *in uncertainties*: John Keats in a letter to his brothers Tom and George dated 22 December 1817, *Letters of John Keats to His Family and Friends*, London, Macmillan, 1925, p. 48.

262 *What you call death* and *Life is your hospital*: Ted Hughes, *Alcestis*, op. cit., pp. 6–7.

263 *that friendship which grows out of love*: Roberto Calasso, *The Marriage of Cadmus and Harmony*, op. cit., p. 73.

263 Kazuo Ishiguro, *Never Let Me Go*, London, Faber & Faber, 2005.

265 *unintelligible ravings ... admirably clear*: Philip Ball, *The Devil's Doctor. Paracelsus and the World of Renaissance Magic and Science*, London, William Heinemann, 2006, p. 190.

265 *his vision of nature was so grand*: Ibid.

265 *man's original and specific mission*: Jolande Jacobi, *Paracelsus. His Life and Work*, in *Paracelsus. Selected Writings*, edited by Jolande Jacobi, London, Routledge & Kegan Paul, 1951, p. 48.

266 *all men and women*: John Paul II, *Letter to Artists*, Vatican, Libreria Editrice Vaticana, 1999.

266 *As bees collect honey*: Rainer Maria Rilke, *Letters to a Young Poet*, op. cit., p. 374.

CONJUNCTION

269 *My eye does not perceive features or details*: Francisco Goya, quoted in A. Arno, *Ostatnie prace Goyi we Frick Collection, czyli portret artysty w późnym wieku* ("Goya's Final Works in the Frick Collection, or a Portrait of the Artist as an Old Man"), "Zeszyty Literackie" 2006, No. 2, pp. 191–193.

269 curandero ... matasanos: Robert Hughes, *Goya*, New York, Knopf, 2003, p. 374.

270 *His embrace is stronger than the grip of death*: A. Arno, op. cit.

270 *As for a plant's growing on trees*: Theophrastus, *De Causis Plantarum*, II, 17.4–5, translated by Benedict Einarson and George K.K. Link, Cambridge, Harvard University Press, 1976, Vol. 1, p. 339.

271 *And so this microscopic organism*: January Weiner, *Życie i ewolucja biosfery. Podręcznik ekologii ogólnej* ("The Life and Evolution of the Biosphere. A General Ecology Handbook"), Warsaw, PWN, 2003, p. 387.

273 *the most important thing*: Andrzej Białas, *Najważniejsze jest odkrywanie praw fundamentalnych* ("The Most Important Thing Is to Discover Basic Laws") in *Po drogach uczonych. Z członkami Polskiej Akademii Umiejętności rozmawia Andrzej Kobos* ("On Learned Paths. Andrzej Kobos in Conversation with Members of the Polish Academy of Arts and Sciences"), Vol. 1, Krakow, PAU, 2007, p. 40.

276 On the gypsy kings: after the First World War "the institution of gypsy kings was revived in Poland. Gypsies of the Kwiek family, who belong to the Kalderari group, have proclaimed themselves successive kings" (from Adam Bartosz, *Cyganie. Historia i kultura* ("The Gypsies, Their History and Culture"), www.muzeum.tarnow.pl/cyganie/przewodnik_rom.html.

276 *it's simply a matter*: Gabriel García Márquez, *One Hundred Years of Solitude*, translated by Gregory Rabassa, London, Jonathan Cape, 1970, p. 2.

276 *as if a gate had been left open*: Seamus Heaney, *Tall Dames*, in *District and Circle*, London, Faber & Faber, 2006, p. 38.

278 *would become a purchaser*: G. Kevin Donovan, *The Physician-Patient Relationship*, in *The Health Care Professional as Friend and Healer*, edited by David C. Thomasma and Judith Lee Kissell, Washington, Georgetown University Press, 2000, p. 19.

278 *It builds a sphere of safety for the patient*: Tadeusz Biesaga, *Elementy etyki lekarskiej* ("Elements of Medical Ethics"), Krakow, Medycyna Praktyczna, 2006, p. 177.

279 *Man is not an aggregate*: Bronisław Wildstein, *Godność umierania i ludzkiego życia* ("The Dignity of Dying and Human Life"), op. cit., p. 17.

280 *consisting of nine elaborate sentences*: Eugeniusz J. Kucharz, *"Przysięga Hipokratesa." Komentarz i nowy przekład na język polski* ("'The Hippocratic Oath'. A Commentary and New Translation into Polish"), "Polskie Archiwum Medycyny Wewnętrznej" 2006, Vol. 116, p. 1099.

281 *We should be hearing*: Sister Małgorzata Chmielewska, *Święty nie prosi o śmierć* ("A Saint Never Asks for Death"), "Dziennik," 2 March 2007, p. 27.

282 *I can talk*: Ibid.

282 *for God's sake*: Ibid.

282 *an ethical perversion*: Tadeusz Biesaga, *Elementy etyki lekarskiej*, op. cit., p. 177.

284 *SCN9A, also known as Nav 1.7*: James J. Cox et al., *An SCN9A Channelopathy Causes Congenital Inability to Experience Pain*, "Nature" 2006, Vol. 444, p. 894.

286 *immortal chicken heart*: See Hannah Landecker, *Culturing Life. How Cells Became Technologies*, Cambridge, Harvard University Press, 2007.

289 *the positivists' paradise has proved empty*: Zbigniew Herbert, *Poeta wobec współczesności* ("The Poet Facing Modernity") in *Wiersze wybrane* ("Selected Poems"), Kraków, Wydawnictwo a5, 2005, p. 398.

290 *Second Life*: Edwin Morgan, *Poetry and Virtual Realities*, in *Contemporary Poetry and Contemporary Science*, edited by Robert Crawford, Oxford, Oxford University Press, 2006, p. 43.